Multi-Energy CT: The New Frontier in Imaging

Editors

SAVVAS NICOLAOU
MOHAMMED F. MOHAMMED

RADIOLOGIC CLINICS OF NORTH AMERICA

www.radiologic.theclinics.com

Consulting Editor
FRANK H. MILLER

July 2018 • Volume 56 • Number 4

ELSEVIER

1600 John F. Kennedy Boulevard • Suite 1800 • Philadelphia, Pennsylvania, 19103-2899

http://www.theclinics.com

RADIOLOGIC CLINICS OF NORTH AMERICA Volume 56, Number 4
July 2018 ISSN 0033-8389, ISBN 13: 978-0-323-61070-4

Editor: John Vassallo (j.vassallo@elsevier.com)
Developmental Editor: Donald Mumford

© **2018 Elsevier Inc. All rights reserved.**

This periodical and the individual contributions contained in it are protected under copyright by Elsevier, and the following terms and conditions apply to their use:

Photocopying

Single photocopies of single articles may be made for personal use as allowed by national copyright laws. Permission of the Publisher and payment of a fee is required for all other photocopying, including multiple or systematic copying, copying for advertising or promotional purposes, resale, and all forms of document delivery. Special rates are available for educational institutions that wish to make photocopies for non-profit educational classroom use. For information on how to seek permission visit www.elsevier.com/permissions or call: (+44) 1865 843830 (UK)/(+1) 215 239 3804 (USA).

Derivative Works

Subscribers may reproduce tables of contents or prepare lists of articles including abstracts for internal circulation within their institutions. Permission of the Publisher is required for resale or distribution outside the institution. Permission of the Publisher is required for all other derivative works, including compilations and translations (please consult www.elsevier.com/permissions).

Electronic Storage or Usage

Permission of the Publisher is required to store or use electronically any material contained in this periodical, including any article or part of an article (please consult www.elsevier.com/permissions). Except as outlined above, no part of this publication may be reproduced, stored in a retrieval system or transmitted in any form or by any means, electronic, mechanical, photocopying, recording or otherwise, without prior written permission of the Publisher.

Notice

No responsibility is assumed by the Publisher for any injury and/or damage to persons or property as a matter of products liability, negligence or otherwise, or from any use or operation of any methods, products, instructions or ideas contained in the material herein. Because of rapid advances in the medical sciences, in particular, independent verification of diagnoses and drug dosages should be made.

Although all advertising material is expected to conform to ethical (medical) standards, inclusion in this publication does not constitute a guarantee or endorsement of the quality or value of such product or of the claims made of it by its manufacturer.

Radiologic Clinics of North America (ISSN 0033-8389) is published bimonthly by Elsevier Inc., 360 Park Avenue South, New York, NY 10010-1710. Months of issue are January, March, May, July, September, and November. Periodicals postage paid at New York, NY and additional mailing offices. Subscription prices are USD 493 per year for US individuals, USD 889 per year for US institutions, USD 100 per year for US students and residents, USD 573 per year for Canadian individuals, USD 1136 per year for Canadian institutions, USD 680 per year for international individuals, USD 1136 per year for international institutions, and USD 315 per year for Canadian and international students/residents. To receive student and resident rate, orders must be accompanied by name of affiliated institution, date of term and the signature of program/residency coordinatior on institution letterhead. Orders will be billed at individual rate until proof of status is received. Foreign air speed delivery is included in all *Clinics* subscription prices. All prices are subject to change without notice. **POSTMASTER:** Send address changes to *Radiologic Clinics of North America*, Elsevier Health Sciences Division, Subscription Customer Service, 3251 Riverport Lane, Maryland Heights, MO63043. **Customer Service: Telephone: 1-800-654-2452** (U.S. and Canada); **1-314-447-8871** (outside U.S. and Canada). **Fax: 1-314-447-8029. E-mail: journalscustomerservice-usa@ elsevier.com (for print support); journalsonlinesupport-usa@elsevier.com (for online support).**

Reprints. For copies of 100 or more of articles in this publication, please contact the Commercial Reprints Department, Elsevier Inc., 360 Park Avenue South, New York, New York 10010-1710. Tel.: +1-212-633-3874; Fax: +1-212-633-3820; E-mail: reprints@elsevier.com.

Radiologic Clinics of North America also published in Greek Paschalidis Medical Publications, Athens, Greece.

Radiologic Clinics of North America is covered in *MEDLINE/PubMed (Index Medicus), EMBASE/Excerpta Medica, Current Contents/Life Sciences, Current Contents/Clinical Medicine, RSNA Index to Imaging Literature, BIOSIS, Science Citation Index,* and *ISI/BIOMED.*

Contributors

CONSULTING EDITOR

FRANK H. MILLER, MD
Chief, Body Imaging Section and Fellowship
Program, Medical Director of MRI, Professor,
Department of Radiology, Northwestern
University Feinberg School of Medicine,
Chicago, Illinois, USA

EDITORS

SAVVAS NICOLAOU, MD
Professor of Radiology, Vice Academic Chair
of Undergraduate Education and CPD, Director
of Emergency/Trauma Imaging, Vancouver
General Hospital, University of British
Columbia, Vancouver, British Columbia,
Canada

MOHAMMED F. MOHAMMED, MBBS, CIIP
Consultant Radiologist, Abdominal Imaging
and Emergency/Trauma Imaging, Medical
Imaging Department, Ministry of the National
Guard, Health Affairs, King Saud bin Abdulaziz
University for Health Sciences, King Abdullah
International Medical Research Center,
Ar Rimayah, Riyadh, Saudi Arabia

AUTHORS

MORITZ H. ALBRECHT, MD
Department of Radiology and Radiological
Science, Division of Cardiovascular
Imaging, Medical University of South
Carolina, Charleston, South Carolina, USA;
Department of Diagnostic and Interventional
Radiology, University Hospital Frankfurt,
Germany

GHASSAN ALMAZIED, MBBS
Medical Imaging Department, Abdominal
Imaging Section, Ministry of the National
Guard, Health Affairs, King Saud bin Abdulaziz
University for Health Sciences, King Abdullah
International Medical Research Center,
Riyadh, Saudi Arabia

LAKSHMI ANANTHAKRISHNAN, MD
Assistant Professor, Department of
Radiology, University of Texas
Southwestern Medical Center, Dallas,
Texas, USA

FAHAD AZZUMEA, MBBS
Medical Imaging Department, Abdominal
Imaging Section, Ministry of the National
Guard, Health Affairs, King Saud bin Abdulaziz
University for Health Sciences, King Abdullah
International Medical Research Center,
Riyadh, Saudi Arabia

DAMIANO CARUSO, MD
Department of Radiological Sciences,
Oncology and Pathology, University of Rome
"Sapienza," Rome, Italy

CARLO N. DE CECCO, MD, PhD
Department of Radiology and Radiological
Science, Division of Cardiovascular Imaging,
Medical University of South Carolina,
Charleston, South Carolina, USA

PATRICIA M. DE GROOT, MD
Associate Professor of Radiology, Department
of Diagnostic Radiology, The University of
Texas MD Anderson Cancer Center, Houston,
Texas, USA

DOMENICO DE SANTIS, MD
Department of Radiology and Radiological
Science, Division of Cardiovascular Imaging,
Medical University of South Carolina,
Charleston, South Carolina, USA; Department
of Radiological Sciences, Oncology and
Pathology, University of Rome "Sapienza,"
Rome, Italy

CIHAN DURAN, MD
Assistant Professor of Radiology, Department
of Diagnostic Radiology, The University of
Texas Medical Branch, Galveston, Texas, USA

MARWEN EID, MD
Department of Radiology and Radiological
Science, Division of Cardiovascular Imaging,
Medical University of South Carolina,
Charleston, South Carolina, USA

KHALED Y. ELBANNA, FRCR
Department of Medical Imaging, Emergency
and Trauma Radiology Division, Sunnybrook
Health Sciences Centre, University of Toronto,
Toronto, Ontario, Canada

MYRNA C. GODOY, MD, PhD
Associate Professor of Radiology, Department
of Diagnostic Radiology, The University of
Texas MD Anderson Cancer Center, Houston,
Texas, USA

BRIAN E. JACOBS, BS
Department of Radiology and Radiological
Science, Division of Cardiovascular Imaging,
Medical University of South Carolina,
Charleston, South Carolina, USA

AVINASH KAMBADAKONE, MD, DNB, FRCR
Assistant Professor, Department of Radiology,
Harvard Medical School, Massachusetts
General Hospital, Boston, Massachusetts, USA

FAISAL KHOSA, MD
Department of Radiology, Vancouver General
Hospital, Vancouver, British Columbia, Canada

BERNHARD KRAUSS, PhD
HC DI CT R&D CTC SA, Siemens Healthcare
GmbH, Forchheim, Germany

ANDREA LAGHI, MD
Department of Radiological Sciences,
Oncology and Pathology, University of Rome
"Sapienza," Rome, Italy

FRANCESCO MACRI, MD, PhD
Research Fellow, Department of Radiology,
Abdominal Imaging Division, Massachusetts
General Hospital, Boston, Massachusetts,
USA; Senior Consultant, Department of
Radiology, University Hospital of Nimes,
Nimes, France

DANIELE MARIN, MD
Associate Professor, Department of Radiology,
Division of Abdominal Imaging, Duke
University, Durham, North Carolina, USA

ALEC J. MEGIBOW, MD, MPH, FACR
Professor of Radiology and Surgery,
Department of Radiology, NYU Langone
Medical Center, New York, New York, USA

ABDELAZIM M.E. MOHAMMED, MBBS
Medical Imaging Department, Abdominal
Imaging Section, Ministry of the National
Guard, Health Affairs, King Saud bin Abdulaziz
University for Health Sciences, King Abdullah
International Medical Research Center,
Riyadh, Saudi Arabia

MOHAMMED F. MOHAMMED, MBBS, CIIP
Consultant Radiologist, Abdominal
Imaging and Emergency/Trauma Imaging,
Medical Imaging Department, Ministry of
the National Guard, Health Affairs, King
Saud bin Abdulaziz University for Health
Sciences, King Abdullah International
Medical Research Center, Ar Rimayah, Riyadh,
Saudi Arabia

DESIREE E. MORGAN, MD
Professor and Vice Chair for Education,
Department of Radiology, The University of
Alabama at Birmingham, Birmingham,
Alabama, USA

NICOLAS MURRAY, MD
Department of Radiology, Vancouver
General Hospital, Vancouver, British Columbia,
Canada

SAVVAS NICOLAOU, MD
Professor of Radiology, Vice Academic Chair
of Undergraduate Education and CPD, Director
of Emergency/Trauma Imaging, Vancouver
General Hospital, University of British
Columbia, Vancouver, British Columbia,
Canada

ERIKA G. ODISIO, MD
Radiology Fellow, Department of Diagnostic Radiology, The University of Texas MD Anderson Cancer Center, Houston, Texas, USA

ANUSHRI PARAKH, MD
Research Fellow, Department of Radiology, Abdominal Imaging Division, Massachusetts General Hospital, Boston, Massachusetts, USA

BHAVIK N. PATEL, MD, MBA
Assistant Professor, Department of Radiology, Division of Abdominal Imaging, Stanford University School of Medicine, Stanford, California, USA

DUSHYANT SAHANI, MD
Assistant Professor, Department of Radiology, Abdominal Imaging Division, Massachusetts General Hospital, Boston, Massachusetts, USA

UWE JOSEPH SCHOEPF, MD
Department of Radiology and Radiological Science, Division of Cardiovascular Imaging, Medical University of South Carolina, Charleston, South Carolina, USA

SAMAD SHAH, MD
Department of Radiology, Vancouver General Hospital, Vancouver, British Columbia, Canada

AARON D. SODICKSON, MD, PhD
Associate Professor, Department of Radiology, Division of Emergency Radiology, Brigham and Women's Hospital, Harvard Medical School, Boston, Massachusetts, USA

CHRISTIAN TESCHE, MD
Department of Radiology and Radiological Science, Division of Cardiovascular Imaging, Medical University of South Carolina, Charleston, South Carolina, USA; Department of Cardiology and Intensive Care Medicine, Heart Center Munich-Bogenhausen, Munich, Germany

MYLENE T. TRUONG, MD
Professor of Radiology, Department of Diagnostic Radiology, The University of Texas MD Anderson Cancer Center, Houston, Texas, USA

AKOS VARGA-SZEMES, MD, PhD
Department of Radiology and Radiological Science, Division of Cardiovascular Imaging, Medical University of South Carolina, Charleston, South Carolina, USA

FRANCES WALSTRA, MD
Department of Radiology, Vancouver General Hospital, Vancouver, British Columbia, Canada

WILLIAM D. WONG, BSC
Department of Radiology, Vancouver General Hospital, Vancouver, British Columbia, Canada

JEREMY R. WORTMAN, MD
Instructor, Department of Radiology, Division of Emergency Radiology, Brigham and Women's Hospital, Harvard Medical School, Boston, Massachusetts, USA

Contents

Dual-Energy Computed Tomography: Technology and Challenges

Bernhard Krauss

Dual-energy computed tomography (CT) is an imaging technique in which the same axial slice of the patient is scanned with two different X-ray spectra to extract chemical information or improve diagnostic image quality. This method is useful for the detection or visualization of heavy atoms, such as iodine, but the differentiation of soft tissue types containing only light atoms is usually not markedly improved compared with single-energy CT. The commercially available dual-energy CT scanners use different technologic approaches that differ in complexity and result quality.

Dual-Energy Computed Tomography: Image Acquisition, Processing, and Workflow

Alec J. Megibow, Avinash Kambadakone, and Lakshmi Ananthakrishnan

Dual-energy computed tomography has been available for more than 10 years; however, it is currently on the cusp of widespread clinical use. The way dual-energy data are acquired and assembled must be appreciated at the clinical level so that the various reconstruction types can extend their diagnostic power. The type of scanner that is present in a given practice dictates the way in which the dual-energy data can be presented and used. This article compares and contrasts how dual source, rapid kilovolt switching, and spectral technologies acquire and present dual-energy reconstructions to practicing radiologists.

Dual-Energy Computed Tomography in Cardiothoracic Vascular Imaging

Domenico De Santis, Marwen Eid, Carlo N. De Cecco, Brian E. Jacobs, Moritz H. Albrecht, Akos Varga-Szemes, Christian Tesche, Damiano Caruso, Andrea Laghi, and Uwe Joseph Schoepf

Dual-energy computed tomography is becoming increasingly widespread in clinical practice. It can expand on the traditional density-based data achievable with single-energy computed tomography by adding novel applications to help reach a more accurate diagnosis. The implementation of this technology in cardiothoracic vascular imaging allows for improved image contrast, metal artifact reduction, generation of virtual unenhanced images, virtual calcium subtraction techniques, cardiac and pulmonary perfusion evaluation, and plaque characterization. The improved diagnostic performance afforded by dual-energy computed tomography is not associated with an increased radiation dose. This article provides an overview of dual-energy computed tomography cardiothoracic vascular applications.

Role of Dual-Energy Computed Tomography in Thoracic Oncology

Erika G. Odisio, Mylene T. Truong, Cihan Duran, Patricia M. de Groot, and Myrna C. Godoy

Dual-energy computed tomography (DECT) is an emerging technology that has potential to enhance diagnostic performance and radiologists' confidence in the evaluation of thoracic malignancies. DECT clinical applications include characterization of solitary pulmonary nodule, lung masses, and mediastinal tumors. DECT-derived iodine uptake quantification may assist in the characterization of tumor differentiation and gene expression. The use of DECT in oncology has potential to improve lung cancer staging, therapy planning, and assessment of response to therapy, as well as detection of incidental pulmonary embolism.

With new developments in workflow automation, as well as technologic advances enabling faster imaging with improved image quality and dose profile, dual-energy computed tomography is being used more often in the imaging of the acutely ill and injured patient. Its ability to identify iodine, differentiate it from hematoma or calcification, and improve contrast resolution has proven invaluable in the assessment of organ perfusion, organ injury, and inflammation.

The added value and strength of dual-energy computed tomography for the evaluation of oncologic patients revolve around the use of lower-energy reconstructed images and iodine material density images. Lower kiloelectron volt simulated monoenergetic images optimize soft tissue tumor to nontumoral attenuation differences and increase contrast to noise ratios to improve lesion detection. Iodine material density images or maps are helpful from a qualitative standpoint for image interpretation because they result in improved detection and characterization of tumors and lymph node involvement and from a quantitative assessment by enabling interrogation of specific properties of tissues to predict and assess therapeutic response.

Dual-energy computed tomography (DECT) is a rapidly growing tool in musculoskeletal radiology. It has been validated as an accurate imaging modality for the assessment of gout and bone marrow edema. DECT can be used to reduce metal artifacts. A few studies have shown its ability to calculate bone mineral density and examine pathologic states in tendons and ligaments. Its capacity for material separation suggests its emergence as a technique for arthrography and for the evaluation of intervertebral discs and other inflammatory arthropathies.

Evolution in computed tomography technology and image reconstruction have significantly changed practice. Dual-energy computed tomography is being increasingly adopted owing to benefits of material separation, quantification, and improved contrast to noise ratio. The radiation dose can match that from single-energy computed tomography. Spectral information derived from a polychromatic x-ray beam at different energies yields in image reconstructions that reduce the number of phases in a multiphasic examination and decrease the absolute amount of contrast media. This increased analytical and image processing capability provides new avenues for addressing radiation dose and iodine exposure concerns.

Dual-energy computed tomography (DECT) is an exciting technology that is increasing in routine use and has the potential for significant clinical impact. With the advancement of DECT, it is important for radiologists to be aware of potential challenges with DECT acquisition and postprocessing and to have a basic knowledge of unique artifacts and diagnostic pitfalls that can occur when interpreting DECT scans and DECT postprocessed images. This article serves as a practical overview of potential problems and diagnostic pitfalls associated with DECT and steps that can be taken to avoid them.

Dual-energy computed tomography (DECT) offers several advantages over conventional single-energy computed tomography. These advantages include improved image quality, beam hardening correction, and metal artifact reduction. In addition, DECT allows derivation of quantitative information through material decomposition analysis. Although newer third-generation rapid-kilovolt switching and dual-source DECT scanners have significantly improved in image quality and workflow compared with initial iterations and early scanners, sources of potential image quality degradation can exist secondary to the inherent capabilities in which the image acquisition occurs.

PROGRAM OBJECTIVE

The objective of the *Radiologic Clinics of North America* is to keep practicing radiologists and radiology residents up to date with current clinical practice in radiology by providing timely articles reviewing the state of the art in patient care.

TARGET AUDIENCE

Practicing radiologists, radiology residents, and other healthcare professionals who provide patient care utilizing radiologic findings.

LEARNING OBJECTIVES

Upon completion of this activity, participants will be able to:
1. Review dual energy CT in cardiothoracic vascular imaging.
2. Discuss strategies to improve image quality on DECT.
3. Recognize advanced muculoskeletal applications of dual-energy CT.

ACCREDITATION

The Elsevier Office of Continuing Medical Education (EOCME) is accredited by the Accreditation Council for Continuing Medical Education (ACCME) to provide continuing medical education for physicians.

The EOCME designates this enduring material for a maximum of 15 *AMA PRA Category 1 Credit*(s)™. Physicians should claim only the credit commensurate with the extent of their participation in the activity.

All other healthcare professionals requesting continuing education credit for this enduring material will be issued a certificate of participation.

DISCLOSURE OF CONFLICTS OF INTEREST

The EOCME assesses conflict of interest with its instructors, faculty, planners, and other individuals who are in a position to control the content of CME activities. All relevant conflicts of interest that are identified are thoroughly vetted by EOCME for fair balance, scientific objectivity, and patient care recommendations. EOCME is committed to providing its learners with CME activities that promote improvements or quality in healthcare and not a specific proprietary business or a commercial interest.

The planning committee, staff, authors and editors listed below have identified no financial relationships or relationships to products or devices they or their spouse/life partner have with commercial interest related to the content of this CME activity:

Ghassan Almazied, MBBS; Lakshmi Ananthakrishnan, MD; Fahad Azzumea, MBBS; Damiano Caruso, MD; Patricia M. de Groot, MD; Domenico De Santis, MD; Cihan Duran, MD; Marwen Eid, MD; Khaled Y. Elbanna, FRCR; Brian E. Jacobs, BS; Avinash Kambadakone, MD, DNB, FRCR; Alison Kemp; Faisal Khosa, MD; Pradeep Kuttysankaran; Andrea Laghi, MD; Francesco Macri, MD, PhD; Frank H. Miller, MD; Abdelazim M.E. Mohammed, MBBS; Mohammed F. Mohammed, MBBS, CIIP; Nicolas Murray, MD; Savvas Nicolaou, MD; Erika G. Odisio, MD; Anushri Parakh, MD; Dushyant Sahani, MD; Samad Shah, MD; Christian Tesche, MD; Mylene T. Truong, MD; John Vassallo; Frances Walstra, MD; William D. Wong, BSC; Jeremy R. Wortman, MD.

The planning committee, staff, authors and editors listed below have identified financial relationships or relationships to products or devices they or their spouse/life partner have with commercial interest related to the content of this CME activity:

Moritz H. Albrecht, MD: has served on a speaker's burea for Siemens Healthcare GmbH.
Carlo N. De Cecco, MD, PhD: has received research support from Siemens Healthcare GmbH and has participated in speaker's bureau for Bayer AG.
Myrna C. Godoy, MD, PhD: has received research support from Siemens Healthcare GmbH.
Bernhard Krauss, PhD: is employed by Siemens Healthcare GmbH.
Daniele Marin, MD: has served on a speaker's bureau, been a consultant/advisor and has received research support from Siemens Healthcare GmbH.
Alec J. Megibow, MD, MPH, FACR: has been a consultant/advisor for Bracco Diagnostic Inc.
Desiree E. Morgan, MD: has received research support from General Electric Company.
Bhavik N. Patel, MD, MBA: has served on a speakers' bureau for General Electric Company.
Uwe Joseph Schoepf, MD: has received research support from Astellas Pharma US, Inc., Bayer AG, General Electric Company, and Siemens Healthcare GmbH; has been a consultant/advisor for the Guerbet Group and has participated in a speaker's burea for HeartFlow, Inc.
Aaron D. Sodickson, MD, PhD: has been a consultant/advisor for and received research support from Siemens Healthcare GmbH, Inc and has been a consultant/advisor for Bayer AG.
Akos Varga-Szemes, MD, PhD: has received research support from Siemens Healthcare GmbH.

UNAPPROVED/OFF-LABEL USE DISCLOSURE

The EOCME requires CME faculty to disclose to the participants:
1. When products or procedures being discussed are off-label, unlabelled, experimental, and/or investigational (not US Food and Drug Administration [FDA] approved); and

2. Any limitations on the information presented, such as data that are preliminary or that represent ongoing research, interim analyses, and/or unsupported opinions. Faculty may discuss information about pharmaceutical agents that is outside of FDA-approved labelling. This information is intended solely for CME and is not intended to promote off-label use of these medications. If you have any questions, contact the medical affairs department of the manufacturer for the most recent prescribing information.

TO ENROLL

To enroll in the *Radiologic Clinics of North America* Continuing Medical Education program, call customer service at 1-800-654-2452 or sign up online at http://www.theclinics.com/home/cme. The CME program is available to subscribers for an additional annual fee of USD 327.60.

METHOD OF PARTICIPATION

In order to claim credit, participants must complete the following:

1. Complete enrolment as indicated above.
2. Read the activity.
3. Complete the CME Test and Evaluation. Participants must achieve a score of 70% on the test. All CME Tests and Evaluations must be completed online.

CME INQUIRIES/SPECIAL NEEDS

For all CME inquiries or special needs, please contact elsevierCME@elsevier.com.

RADIOLOGIC CLINICS OF NORTH AMERICA

THE CLINICS ARE AVAILABLE ONLINE!
Access your subscription at:
www.theclinics.com

Dedications

From Dr Mohammed: To Ghada and Jana.

From Dr Nicolaou: I dedicate this special project to my supportive, lovely, beautiful wife, Sonya, to my deceased son, Lazarus, to my deceased father, Charalambous, to my mother, Androulla for her undying loyalty, and to my brothers, Nick and George, for their mentorship loyalty and guidance.

Radiol Clin N Am 56 (2018) xiii
https://doi.org/10.1016/j.rcl.2018.06.001
0033-8389/18/© 2018 Published by Elsevier Inc.

Preface

Multienergy Computed Tomography: A New Horizon in Computed Tomographic Imaging

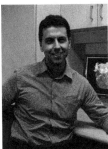

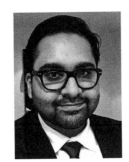

Savvas Nicolaou, MD   Mohammed F. Mohammed, MBBS, CIIP

Editors

Radiology has always been at the forefront of technological advances in medicine. Although first conceptualized in 1979, multienergy computed tomography (CT) became practically feasible only recently, when technological limitations were addressed. The first multienergy CT scanner was released in 2006 and utilized two separate x-ray tubes offset by 90°, which enabled simultaneously scanning at two different energy levels. This unique design allowed radiologists to exploit the differences in attenuation of various tissues within the body in order to identify their composition. Further introduction of other new technologies allowed for rapid kilovoltage switching, and sandwich detectors capable of registering low and high kilovolts from a single polychromatic beam also capitalized on the principle of scanning at different energy levels.

These CT technological advances have opened the door to new and exciting clinical applications in medical imaging. Early clinical uses included material characterization of renal stones, in which multienergy CT could help differentiate between calcium oxalate and uric acid stones, through material labeling and assigning different color coding to help differentiate them. Multienergy CT has been validated for the detection and diagnosis of gout, where uric acid deposits could be accurately identified in and around joints. Through a unique three-material decomposition algorithm, we can now subtract iodine or calcium from images to create virtual noncontrast images/virtual calcium subtracted data that allow one to quantify the amount of iodine in one voxel or reveal the presence of bone marrow edema in tubular bones. This opens up numerous applications for bowel ischemia, oncologic applications to assess for malignancy or increase lesion conspicuity, for perfused blood volume imaging to interrogate organ perfusion, and for the presence of bone marrow edema in the presence of subtle nondisplaced fractures.

There has been much research undertaken in order to take advantage of this technology, which continues to find applications in many aspects of radiology, including in cardiovascular, abdominal, thoracic, musculoskeletal, vascular, and neurologic imaging. Many of these applications are explored in this issue of *Radiologic Clinics of North America.*

In addition, the two-detector design of dual-source multienergy CT scanners has allowed for dramatic increases in temporal resolution when scanned at the same energy level, which has allowed for improved imaging of structures most often susceptible to motion, including the heart and thoracic vasculature. Advances in

Radiol Clin N Am 56 (2018) xv–xvi
https://doi.org/10.1016/j.rcl.2018.04.001
0033-8389/18/© 2018 Published by Elsevier Inc.

postprocessing algorithms have allowed advances to be made in radiation dose reduction in multienergy imaging.

In this issue, we introduce the reader to the physics and technology behind multienergy CT, image acquisition techniques and workflow tips, clinical applications of multienergy CT, and common problems and pitfalls that may arise during multienergy CT imaging and potential solutions. We hope that this issue will be informative and provide case examples of how multienergy CT can enrich your practice as well as help problem solve challenging cases.

Ultimately it is our patients and our referring clinicians who will benefit from this technology as this issue illustrates through many examples on the clinical impact of improved patient care and management that can be achieved in a new world of imaging with a multitude of bright colors with multienergy CT.

Savvas Nicolaou, MD
Emergency/Trauma Imaging
Vancouver General Hospital
University of British Columbia
899 West 12th Avenue
Vancouver, British Columbia V5Z1M9, Canada

Mohammed F. Mohammed, MBBS, CIIP
Abdominal Imaging and Emergency/
Trauma Imaging
Ministry of the National Guard, Health Affairs
Medical Imaging Department
Prince Mutib Ibn Abdullah
Ibn Abdulaziz Road
Ar Rimayah, Riyadh 14611, Saudi Arabia

E-mail addresses:
Savvas.Nicolaou@vch.ca (S. Nicolaou)
mohammed.f.mohammed@gmail.com
(M.F. Mohammed)

Dual-Energy Computed Tomography
Technology and Challenges

Bernhard Krauss, PhD

KEYWORDS

• Dual-energy CT • Spectral CT • Spectral imaging • CT technology • Material differentiation

KEY POINTS

- Dual-energy computed tomography (CT) or spectral CT can be used to detect, visualize, quantify or subtract materials with a high atomic number, such as calcium, iron or iodine.
- At the same time, conventional CT images using the whole radiation dose can be generated.
- Scanner types differ in material differentiation quality, robustness against patient motion, and radiation dose efficiency.
- Material differentiation depends on lesion size and image noise, and may be impossible if the X-ray attenuation of the candidate materials is similar for both spectra.

THE CLINICAL APPLICABILITY OF DUAL-ENERGY COMPUTED TOMOGRAPHY

With traditional computed tomography (CT) scanners, the evaluation of clinical CT images is mainly based on the morphologic information, which results from the different X-ray attenuation of neighboring tissues. Relevant pathologic states are indicated by abnormalities in shape or texture, whereas X-ray attenuation of suspicious areas is often only qualitatively assessed in terms of being hypodense, hyperdense, or isodense with respect to the surrounding material. In clinical routine, the X-ray attenuation itself is only evaluated in selected cases. For example, quantitative CT (QCT) can be used for the measurement of bone mineral density in the spine[1] or noncontrast CT can be used for the evaluation of specific soft tissue lesions, such as cysts[2] or adrenal adenomas.[3] However, for materials such as bone or iodine, a problem is that the CT value depends on the used X-ray spectrum, as well as on patient diameter and patient shape in each axial slice. Hence, for example, the measurement of bone mineral density with QCT traditionally requires dedicated scan modes,[4] special patient positioning, and sophisticated evaluation tools.[5]

In this way, single-energy CT is usually semi-quantitative when elements with atomic numbers sufficiently higher than oxygen are involved. Leaving aside practical considerations, this problem could, in theory, be avoided by using a monochromatic synchrotron X-ray source instead of a conventional X-ray tube.[6] With a clinical single-energy CT system this is not possible because the X-ray spectrum originating from the X-ray tube is polychromatic. Because body tissues have a higher attenuation at low X-ray energies than at high X-ray energies, the mean energy of the X-ray spectrum increases with increasing attenuation by the patient. Although this can be compensated for in the case of water-equivalent materials such as soft tissue, there is a remaining beam-hardening effect for the heavier atoms. This leads to the observation that the CT value (in Hounsfield units) of the same small contrast agent sample in air can be 30% higher than inside a realistic abdominal phantom. With larger amounts of bone or iodine, there can also be beam-hardening artifacts, which are seen as

HC DI CT R&D CTC SA, Siemens Healthcare GmbH, Siemensstrasse 3, 91301 Forchheim, Germany
E-mail address: bernhard.krauss@siemens-healthineers.com

Radiol Clin N Am 56 (2018) 497–506
https://doi.org/10.1016/j.rcl.2018.03.008
0033-8389/18/© 2018 Elsevier Inc. All rights reserved.

dark and bright areas in the soft tissue in the vicinity of these materials.

In 1976, it was already noticed[7] that dual-energy CT or spectral CT can be used to avoid this potential problem by allowing for the reconstruction of monoenergetic images without the need for a synchrotron facility. With dual-energy CT, the same axial slice of a patient is (ideally) simultaneously scanned with 2 different X-ray spectra. In this way it is directly possible to calculate images of the water-equivalent density and the contrast agent concentration in milligrams per milliliter from the dual-energy data. In a second step, the images can be merged again to generate monoenergetic images. Although it is obvious that this method will work for water and contrast agent, it is not obvious, instead actually true, that the same approach also works for all other materials with atomic numbers up to iodine.

In practice, the problems with beam hardening turned out to be less relevant than anticipated at that time. Modern multislice CT systems use rather strong X-ray prefiltration, which narrows the original spectrum. In addition, raw data-based, single-energy iterative methods can be used to achieve beam-hardening artifact reduction.[8] This feature is currently commercially available on clinical CT scanners, for example, for improving the image quality of high-dose noncontrast scans of the brain.

However, 3 advantages of monoenergetic images persist. First, reproducible CT values for all materials involving heavier atoms may allow for a more standardized differentiation between certain pathologic or nonpathologic lesions.[9] Second, monoenergetic images at energy levels higher than 100 keV have turned out to be beneficial for reducing beam-hardening artifacts that are associated with metal prostheses of moderate size, such as spine implants,[10] because they also tend to suppress artifacts from scattered radiation.[11,12] The third advantage is that, in combination with modern image noise reduction techniques such as iterative reconstruction, the energy level of a monochromatic image allows for modifying the iodine contrast without scaling image noise by the same factor.[13–15] This means that, in contrast to simple image windowing, the kiloelectron volt level allows for material-specific windowing so that materials become distinguishable or can be visualized with a high apparent contrast to noise ratio (CNR).

There are also caveats to these statements. The first is that iodine uptake at a fixed point in time also depends on effects not related to the scanner, such as injection protocol, cardiac output, and patient blood volume. Hence, monoenergetic images may be objective in terms of the involved X-ray physics but, in some situations, single-energy dynamic scan protocols may actually be more objective in assessing lesion physiology.[16,17] The second is that it is actually very difficult to assess the clinical benefit of advanced image reconstruction or denoising techniques because the widely used CNR-value may not be sufficient to quantify the diagnostic value of the image.[18]

Despite these issues, monoenergetic imaging has been demonstrated to be possibly the most relevant application of dual-energy CT[19,20] and, currently, it is presumably offered on all commercially available dual-energy CT systems.

Probably the second most popular application of dual-energy CT is the selective visualization of iodine contrast agent and the underlying soft tissues,[21–23] which is also called virtual noncontrast imaging. Clearly, the detection of iodine enhancement is also possible with single energy scans with and without contrast agent; however, the advantage of dual-energy CT is that an additional noncontrast CT scan may not always be indicated. It may also not be sufficient if tissue density changes between the 2 scans, which applies, for example, for the evaluation of iodine uptake in lung tissue.[24] Another relevant application of dual-energy CT is for cases in which iodine has already been injected; for example, as part of an angiography examination, so that there is no chance to obtain an additional true noncontrast scan.[25] The question of whether quantitative iodine uptake can be used to distinguish between different lesion types is an active field of research[26,27] and promising results have been obtained so far. It should be noted that the dual-energy approach does not necessarily imply a higher sensitivity for enhancing lesions but it can definitely improve the conspicuity of iodine uptake, as well as enable the differentiation between iodine uptake and, for example, hemorrhagic lesions.

In addition, the detection of heavy materials in the human body can also be extended to other materials, such as diffuse calcium depositions in the brain,[28] silicone in lymph nodes,[29] or iron deposition in the liver.[30] Notably, in these cases, dual-energy CT cannot directly differentiate between the accumulated heavy atoms such as silicon or iodine. Instead, the concentration can often only be calculated using the assumption that the identity of the heavy atom is known. It should be noted that, at the same CT value enhancement, the concentration in milligrams per milliliters of materials with a lower atomic number (e.g., iron) is higher than the concentration of iodine. Hence, iodine concentrations of 0.5 mg/mL may still be detectable with dual-energy CT,[31] whereas the detection threshold for iron has been reported to be 7 mg/g dry tissue, or approximately 2 mg/mL.[32]

Sometimes the diagnostic question is different and, instead of having an unknown concentration of a foreign atom in soft tissue, several material types must be distinguished. This applies, for example, in the case of kidney stones, which can be distinguished by measuring the slope between the measured low-energy and high-energy CT values of the stone and the known low-energy and high-energy CT values of kidney parenchyma. In this way, a binary classification can be made into uric acid stones and nonuric acid stones.[33,34] This approach is known as material labeling. Alternatively, the stone type can also be characterized by calculating the effective atomic number of a material.[35] However, as in the case of concentration measurements, the effective atomic number does not uniquely identify material composition. For example, iodine in vessels and bone can have similar effective atomic number, although their chemical composition is very different.

In conclusion, dual-energy CT is helpful if materials with a higher effective atomic number have to be distinguished, visualized, characterized, quantified, or subtracted. In a hypothetical human body consisting only of the same chemical composition with varying material density, dual-energy CT would be useless.

DUAL-ENERGY COMPUTED TOMOGRAPHY TECHNOLOGY

The quasi-simultaneous acquisition of 2 different X-ray spectra in the same CT scanner faces technical challenges. In contrast to color photography, in which filter materials are placed on top of the active detector elements to generate different spectra from the same incident light, this is not an option for X-ray imaging. The difficulty is that such filter materials would eliminate X-ray photons after the beam has already traversed the patient, so that, effectively, patient dose gets wasted. There are currently 3 approaches to this task: different X-ray spectra are generated by the same X-ray tube, 2 X-ray tubes are used and operated at different voltages, or the detector obtains information about the incident X-ray spectrum.

Historically, the first commercially available dual-energy CT scanner[36] was the SOMATOM DR (Siemens AG, Erlangen, Germany) in the 1980s. This was a single-source dual-energy CT scanner that could rapidly switch the tube voltage between 85 kV and 125 kV so that each detector reading was acquired with a different voltage than its predecessor or follower. However, the term rapid was relative because 1 gantry rotation

of this single-slice sequential mode CT scanner took at least 5 seconds. Therefore, the most important clinical application explored at that time was the measurement of the bone mineral density in the trabecular bone of the vertebral body, which represented pioneering work for bone mineral density measurements.

Currently, clinical dual-energy CT scanners of several different types are commercially available.[37] The most basic implementation can be found on the slow kilovolt-switching scanners, which perform 2 subsequent spiral CT scans at different voltages.[38] Although they offer good spectral resolution, they are more sensitive to patient motion that occurs during or between the 2 CT scans. The problem is greatly alleviated by modern multislice CT scanners that can perform thin-slice acquisitions of the whole abdomen within seconds so that nonrigid registration algorithms[39] can compensate for shifts between images.

Also, other single-source dual-energy techniques have been developed, such as the use of a spectral filter that splits the X-ray beam into a low-energy and a high-energy part in front of the patient,[40] or an interleaved spiral scan, in which the CT value is switched after each rotation.[41] Using wide-area detectors, it is additionally possible to perform 2 subsequent scans with different tube voltages and, in this way, cover a whole organ within 2 rotations.[42] Finally, modern and improved versions of fast kilovolt-switching have been invented.[43]

Dual-energy or spectral CT is also possible with dual-source CT scanners, in which 2 independent tube or detector systems reside within the same gantry and are mounted using an angle of approximately 90°. With this design, fast cardiac imaging and high-pitch single-energy scanning are possible, in addition to dual-energy CT.[44]

Finally, energy sensitive detectors have been introduced. For example, a combination of 2 detector layers of scintillation material can be used to separate spectra because low-energy photons are statistically more frequently absorbed in the top detector layer.[45] On the other hand, a more deterministic separation of low-energy photons and high-energy photons can be achieved by using photon-counting detectors that are not based on scintillator material. For these detectors, heavy semiconductors are used to convert photon energy directly into a charge pulse, so that, in principle, the energy of each photon can be measured individually.[46,47] Current systems of this type are still at the level of research prototypes and it will still take time to develop commercial products.

One difficulty is that each of the presented scanner designs has advantages and disadvantages; it is up to the user to decide which criteria seem to be more important. Hence, a deeper understanding of the involved technologies is useful.

X-RAY SPECTRA AND THEIR IMPACT

When considering dual-energy CT, it is first necessary to appreciate the effects of the X-ray source spectrum, the detector, and the patient who is effectively acting as additional filter material in the X-ray beam. All these components affect the CT values of iodine contrast agent, whereas the CT value of water and water-equivalent materials will, by definition, be independent of the spectrum. Usually a single sample of iodine contrast agent is sufficient to benchmark the spectral behavior of a scanner because the behavior of other materials can be derived from it.[48]

The measured CT value of iodine in the image mainly depends on the energy (E) dependent attenuation coefficient $\mu(E)$ averaged over the X-ray spectrum $S(E)$ that originates from the source and is recorded by the detector.[49] The detected X-ray spectra $S(E)$ for different tube voltages and beam filtrations are shown in **Fig. 1** assuming a typical scintillator-based CT detector and a patient diameter of 35 cm. The spectra are fairly wide, which means that the mean energy of the spectrum does not accurately predict the measured iodine CT value in HU

because of the strong decrease in the contrast attenuation with energy. Instead, the concept of an equivalent monoenergetic energy level can be introduced so that the measured iodine attenuation in Hounsfield units is the same for the polychromatic spectrum and for the monochromatic spectrum at this energy. Typically, an energy level of 70 keV is assumed to be equivalent to a polychromatic spectrum at 120 kV.

Another measurable quantity directly linked to the X-ray spectrum is image noise. Usually, the noise in CT images is due to statistical fluctuations in the number of detected photons, which are unavoidable.[50] The important property of this photon noise is that it does not matter if 1 X-ray exposure is taken at 1 tube current or 2 exposures with the same spectrum are taken with half the tube current and subsequently averaged. Hence, it is also possible to split the dose into 2 different X-ray spectra and reobtain an average image with similar image noise as long as the dose efficiencies of the used spectra are not too dissimilar. However, there are limitations to this. For example, using a tube voltage of 80 kV at 40 cm patient diameter can lead to a very low photon flux at the detector, which means that the resulting image may also show electronics noise. However, this type of noise is not the same if radiation dose is first split into 2 spectra and the images are then merged again. Hence, dual-energy CT may

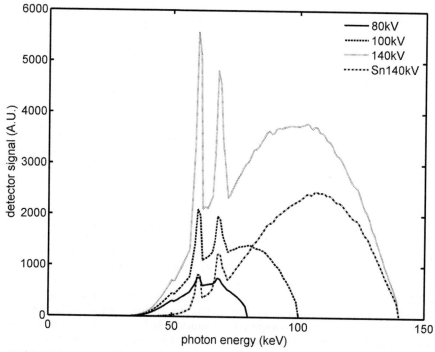

Fig. 1. Detected X-ray spectrum S(E) behind 35 cm of water for commonly used tube voltages with or without additional tin filtration. Photon energy is given in kiloelectron volt (keV), tube voltage is shown in kilovolt (kV), the usage of an additional tin-filter is indicated by the preffix "Sn" in front of the voltage. The detector signal is given in arbitrary units (A.U.).

not be a good option for ultralow dose scanning where electronics noise becomes more important. On the other hand, this limitation naturally disappears for quantum counting detectors, which are assumed to be free from electronics noise.[51]

The third measurable quantity that depends directly on the X-ray spectrum is radiation dose.[52] It is very important to specify how the radiation dose should be measured but for most CT applications it will be sufficient to use the CT dose index ($CTDI_{vol}$) for optimization purposes.

The most important derived quantity for each spectrum is the dose efficiency; that is, the image noise that is obtained at a fixed dose value. Dose efficiency is usually better at low kilovolts for small patient diameters, whereas it is better at 140 kV or 150 kV for large patient diameters.[53] This means that dose efficiency changes with the typical energy of the photon spectrum. On the other hand, the width of the X-ray spectrum also matters because conventional integrating detectors weigh 120 keV photons by a factor of 3 stronger than 40 keV photons, which is not statistically appropriate. Moreover, the low-energy parts of the spectrum tend to be completely absorbed by the patient without contributing to the image. For these reasons, wide spectra can be significantly optimized in terms of dose efficiency by, for example, introducing a tin-filter that transmits

only the high-energy photons but at the cost of increased tube load.[54]

Spectral optimization for dual-energy scanners[55] faces technical boundary constraints. For example, it is not feasible to change X-ray filtration for the whole detector within milliseconds because of the tremendous acceleration values that would be required. Another limitation is that X-ray tube output must be sufficient to image a real patient, which probably excludes very low tube voltages, such as 60 keV, as well as very thick filters, such as greater than 1 mm of tin.

Notably, dual-energy usually also means dual purpose. Each dual-energy scan must guarantee that a conventional diagnostic CT image can be obtained at reasonable radiation dose in addition to an optimal evaluation of the dual-energy information. At the same time, iodine enhancement in this conventional CT image is a relevant parameter. It is known that 120 kV-equivalent mixed images[56,57] can be obtained from different combinations of spectra. Such mixed images are simply calculated as a sum the CT-value in the first image x1 multiplied by a weighting factor w and the CT-value in the second image x2 multiplied by a weighting factor 1-w. The only difference is that for each combination of spectra, image weighting and dose splitting have to be adjusted. However, dual-energy CT is also an option for CT angiography

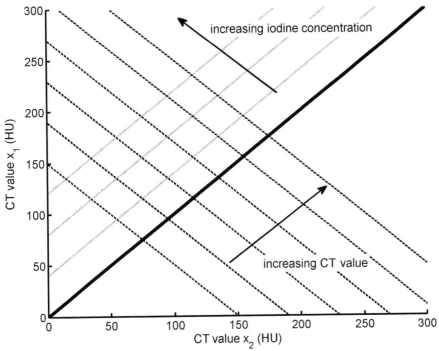

Fig. 2. Relationship between originally measured CT values and the quantities of interest. The CT value at 1 energy is plotted versus the CT value at the other energy. Dashed lines correspond to a fixed CT value in the 120 kV-equivalent image. Dotted lines correspond to a fixed iodine concentration.

scans in which 70kV- or 80kV-equivalent would be preferable because nonlinear image processing allows for selective contrast enhancement in monoenergetic images, as previously described.

In mathematical terms, the dual purpose of dual-energy CT can be expressed by relating the two originally measured CT-values for each voxel to two independent quantities of interest (Fig. 2). Instead of looking at the low-energy and high-energy images separately, the 2 images can be linearly combined to obtain a 120 kV-equivalent mixed image, as well as a difference image $\Delta x = x_{low} - x_{high}$, in which the CT values x_{low} and x_{high} are the respective low-energy and high-energy CT values of the same voxel. For the simple case of a heavy atom such as iodine that is accumulated in water, blood, or soft tissue, Δx is approximately proportional to the concentration of this atom.[58] Clearly, if the high-energy spectrum would measure the limiting value of 0 HU iodine enhancement, this would maximize the CT value difference but at the same time diminish iodine CNR in the mixed image. For this reason, dual-energy CT scan modes will try to balance the image quality of the 2 resulting images, whereas, for cases in which only 1 diagnostic image with specific properties is needed, other approaches can be considered, such as single-energy low-kilovolt imaging[59] or the additional acquisition of a true noncontrast image.

On the other hand it is still true that a large ratio of the iodine enhancement ratio x_{low}/x_{high} is beneficial for dual-energy evaluation.[60] Especially in the context of contrast agent subtraction, it can be shown that this ratio is strongly anticorrelated with the image noise of the remaining virtual noncontrast (VNC) image and tends to reduce systematic uncertainties. Hence, to obtain stable CT values in VNC images, either the iodine enhancement ratio has to be maximized or the scanner calibration has to be carefully optimized so that CT value stability is much better than the sometimes assumed value of plus or minus 5 HU for clinical CT scanners.[61] This may also require countermeasures against radiation that is scattered by the patient and inadvertently hits the detector.[62] In practice, typical accuracies in the order of plus or minus 10 HU have been observed in direct comparisons between true noncontrast and VNC images.[63,64]

TECHNICAL CHALLENGES AND DUAL-ENERGY COMPUTED TOMOGRAPHY

Several technical challenges have shown up in the context of dual-energy CT. One of the first questions was how to handle image noise. As has already been pointed out, image noise in the 120 kV-equivalent monoenergetic or mixed images is not necessarily higher than for standard single-energy CT scans performed at the same radiation dose. However, this is not true for the other output image. Already, for the simple difference between the 2 original low-energy and high-energy images, image noise is higher than in the mixed image by a factor of 2 (assuming same image noise in each image). However, when this image is rescaled to represent true contrast agent enhancement, image noise in Hounsfield units is easily increased by an additional factor of 2 or more. Therefore, the image noise is not a consequence of quantum noise but of noise propagation properties of the algorithm used. Fortunately, the availability of a perfectly registered high-quality prior image allows for substantial denoising of the high-noise iodine image or monoenergetic image.[13] This processing step can be separated from the additional use of iterative reconstruction, which can reduce image noise even further,[65] but on some CT scanners[66,67] both approaches are merged.

For high-precision measurement of the iodine density in the human body, a limitation can be that realistic body materials may not be exactly water-equivalent. For example, subcutaneous and visceral fat show a negative iodine density when starting from the simple difference image. This problem can be avoided by generalizing the analysis to a 3-material or multimaterial decomposition, which explicitly includes fat and soft tissue as base materials.[68] Such a method has, for example, been proposed for use in the liver[69] but it requires that the exact attenuation values of the involved materials must be known.

Temporal resolution is sometimes mentioned as among the key requirements for dual-energy CT but this term is often not precisely defined. Most current dual-energy CT scanners need at least 125 ms (corresponding to 250 ms gantry rotation time) to acquire the minimum amount of raw data needed to reconstruct 1 image, so that motion on this time scale will always lead to sizable motion artifacts. On the other hand, temporal coherence, that is, the displacement between the original low-energy and high-energy information due to motion, depends on the system type and is best for energy-sensitive detectors. Both time scales are relevant for dual-energy imaging. Patient motion is known to lead to raw data inconsistencies so that reconstructed CT values, as well as derived material concentration images, will be systematically wrong on all currently available scanners. This effect is typically seen in quickly moving organs such as heart, lungs, or colon. It is unlikely that problems with temporal resolution can be completely avoided in the future because much faster gantry rotation times would be needed.

Finally, some dual-energy applications are reaching the technical limits of current technology because of low CNR or small lesion size. One example for this is bone marrow imaging, which is a challenging application because calcium and soft tissue have more similar dual-energy behavior than soft tissue and iodine. Although several publications have demonstrated the clinical feasibility of this approach for the extremities and pelvis,[70,71] especially for young patients, the application to spine imaging[72] is hampered by the different bone marrow composition in the vertebrae. Although bone marrow edema is easily seen on the background of yellow marrow, the contrast with respect to red marrow is much smaller. Another challenging case is the base material decomposition into iodine and calcified plaques,[73] which, in principle, allows for the isolation of the vessel lumen. In this case, iodine and calcium are rather similar in their dual-energy attenuation behavior. Furthermore, the relevant structures are extremely small and subject to motion.

FUTURE CHALLENGES

Dual-energy CT can be regarded as a new imaging modality because the diagnostic performance goes dramatically beyond the capabilities of traditional single-energy CT scanners. This can be seen from the tremendous academic impact in recent years (more than 1000 peer reviewed publications), as well as the substantial number of routine CT scans that are performed in dual-energy mode on various scanner types all around the world. Nonetheless, dual-energy CT is sufficiently close to single-energy CT that it can replace a conventional CT scan.

However, there are several issues that can be confusing about dual-energy CT for the first time user. Dual-energy CT is not currently available on all CT scanners and technical implementations can be very different. Current limitations related to scan mode, such as potentially longer scan time, limitations concerning tube current modulation, or the inability to perform spectral scans at low-equivalent kilovolts, must be balanced against the additional information provided. There is no doubt that these practical issues can be solved. Nevertheless, the workflow may currently deviate from the traditional CT workflow. In addition, there is the challenge that the additional information must be transferred, managed, and stored, which means at least a modest increase in PACS load. In this case, it can probably be argued that the trend to also store thin-slice data on the PACS had at least the same impact with respect to the required data traffic. This shows that workflow is certainly an important aspect, along with result quality, and all major vendors are currently offering improved workflow solutions.

Conversely, the speed of the diagnostic workup can actually be improved by the use of dual-energy CT because diagnosis may now be possible in difficult cases. Incidental findings that would otherwise require a patient recall may be addressed using dual-energy CT. Noninvasive tests; for example, for the detection of dense urate or uric acid in the human body, have now become possible. Finally, lesion detection may become easier because of improved conspicuity, thus increasing diagnostic performance.

Dual-energy CT can also be seen as a means to standardize CT image impression independent of the exact technical parameters of the scanning device. One problem with the idea of standardization is that dual-energy CT can only handle spectral differences between scanners. However, there are other factors that have an impact on the measured CT values in a lesion, such as convolution kernel, slice-sensitivity profile, iterative reconstruction, and scattered radiation. This means that, especially for small lesions or large contrasts, spectral scanners may still differ in the observed CT values, even if the same nominal energy level in kiloelectron volts is selected. For this reason, irrespective of all other benefits, dual-energy CT can only be the first step toward a completely standardized viewing of CT images.

REFERENCES

1. Adams JE. Quantitative computed tomography. Eur J Radiol 2009;71(3):415–24.
2. O'Connor SD, Silverman SG, Ip IK, et al. Simple cyst-appearing renal masses at unenhanced CT: can they be presumed to be benign? Radiology 2013;269(3):793–800.
3. Schieda N, Siegelman ES. Update on CT and MRI of adrenal nodules. AJR Am J Roentgenol 2017;208(6): 1206–17.
4. Bligh M, Bidaut L, White RA, et al. Helical multidetector row quantitative computed tomography (QCT) precision. Acad Radiol 2009;16(2):150–9.
5. Klotz E, Kalender WA, Sandor T. Automated definition and evaluation of anatomical ROI's for bone mineral determination by QCT. IEEE Trans Med Imaging 1989;8(4):371–6.
6. Stevenson AW, Hall CJ, Mayo SC, et al. Analysis and interpretation of the first monochromatic X-ray tomography data collected at the Australian Synchrotron Imaging and Medical beamline. J Synchrotron Radiat 2012;19(Pt 5):728–50.

7. Alvarez RE, Macovski A. Energy-selective reconstructions in X-ray computerized tomography. Phys Med Biol 1976;21(5):733–44.

8. Joseph PM, Spital RD. A method for correcting bone induced artifacts in computed tomography scanners. J Comput Assist Tomogr 1978;2(1):100–8.

9. Yu L, Leng S, McCollough CH. Dual-energy CT-based monochromatic imaging. AJR Am J Roentgenol 2012;199(5 Suppl):S9–15.

10. Bamberg F, Dierks A, Nikolaou K, et al. Metal artifact reduction by dual energy computed tomography using monoenergetic extrapolation. Eur Radiol 2011;21(7):1424–9.

11. Huang JY, Kerns JR, Nute JL, et al. An evaluation of three commercially available metal artifact reduction methods for CT imaging. Phys Med Biol 2015;60(3):1047–67.

12. Neuhaus V, Große Hokamp N, Abdullayev N, et al. Metal artifact reduction by dual-layer computed tomography using virtual monoenergetic images. Eur J Radiol 2017;93:143–8.

13. Grant KL, Flohr TG, Krauss B, et al. Assessment of an advanced image-based technique to calculate virtual monoenergetic computed tomographic images from a dual-energy examination to improve contrast-to-noise ratio in examinations using iodinated contrast media. Invest Radiol 2014;49(9):586–92.

14. Fuchs TA, Stehli J, Fiechter M, et al. First experience with monochromatic coronary computed tomography angiography from a 64-slice CT scanner with Gemstone Spectral Imaging (GSI). J Cardiovasc Comput Tomogr 2013;7(1):25–31.

15. Tsang DS, Merchant TE, Merchant SE, et al. Quantifying potential reduction in contrast dose with monoenergetic images synthesized from dual-layer detector spectral CT. Br J Radiol 2017;90:20170290.

16. Thaiss WM, Sauter AW, Bongers M, et al. Clinical applications for dual energy CT versus dynamic contrast enhanced CT in oncology. Eur J Radiol 2015;84(12):2368–79.

17. Gordic S, Puippe GD, Krauss B, et al. Correlation between dual-energy and perfusion CT in patients with hepatocellular carcinoma. Radiology 2016;280(1):78–87.

18. Kofler JM, Yu L, Leng S, et al. Assessment of low-contrast resolution for the American College of Radiology computed tomographic accreditation program: what is the impact of iterative reconstruction? J Comput Assist Tomogr 2015;39(4):619–23.

19. Lenga L, Albrecht MH, Othman AE, et al. Monoenergetic dual-energy computed tomographic imaging: cardiothoracic applications. J Thorac Imaging 2017;32(3):151–8.

20. Marin D, Boll DT, Mileto A, et al. State of the art: dual-energy CT of the abdomen. Radiology 2014;271(2):327–42.

21. Connolly MJ, McInnes MD, El-Khodary M, et al. Diagnostic accuracy of virtual non-contrast enhanced dual-energy CT for diagnosis of adrenal adenoma: a systematic review and meta-analysis. Eur Radiol 2017;27(10):4324–35.

22. Wortman JR, Bunch PM, Fulwadhva UP, et al. Dual-energy CT of incidental findings in the abdomen: can we reduce the need for follow-up imaging? AJR Am J Roentgenol 2016;W1–11. [Epub ahead of print].

23. Agrawal MD, Pinho DF, Kulkarni NM, et al. Oncologic applications of dual-energy CT in the abdomen. Radiographics 2014;34(3):589–612.

24. Remy-Jardin M, Faivre JB, Pontana F, et al. Thoracic applications of dual energy. Semin Respir Crit Care Med 2014;35(1):64–73.

25. Postma AA, Das M, Stadler AA, et al. Dual-energy CT: what the neuroradiologist should know. Curr Radiol Rep 2015;3(5):16.

26. Mileto A, Marin D, Alfaro-Cordoba M, et al. Iodine quantification to distinguish clear cell from papillary renal cell carcinoma at dual-energy multidetector CT: a multireader diagnostic performance study. Radiology 2014;273(3):813–20.

27. Tawfik AM, Razek AA, Kerl JM, et al. Comparison of dual-energy CT-derived iodine content and iodine overlay of normal, inflammatory and metastatic squamous cell carcinoma cervical lymph nodes. Eur Radiol 2014;24(3):574–80.

28. Hu R, Daftari Besheli L, Young J, et al. Dual-energy head CT enables accurate distinction of intraparenchymal hemorrhage from calcification in emergency department patients. Radiology 2016;280(1):177–83.

29. Johnson TR, Himsl I, Hellerhoff K, et al. Dual-energy CT for the evaluation of silicone breast implants. Eur Radiol 2013;23(4):991–6.

30. Luo XF, Yang Y, Yan J, et al. Virtual iron concentration imaging based on dual-energy CT for noninvasive quantification and grading of liver iron content: an iron overload rabbit model study. Eur Radiol 2015;25(9):2657–64.

31. Mileto A, Marin D, Ramirez-Giraldo JC, et al. Accuracy of contrast-enhanced dual-energy MDCT for the assessment of iodine uptake in renal lesions. AJR Am J Roentgenol 2014;202(5):W466–74.

32. Luo XF, Xie XQ, Cheng S, et al. Dual-energy CT for patients suspected of having liver iron overload: can virtual iron content imaging accurately quantify liver iron content? Radiology 2015;277(1):95–103.

33. Qu M, Ramirez-Giraldo JC, Leng S, et al. Dual-energy dual-source CT with additional spectral filtration can improve the differentiation of non-uric acid renal stones: an ex vivo phantom study. AJR Am J Roentgenol 2011;196(6):1279–87.

34. Stolzmann P, Kozomara M, Chuck N, et al. In vivo identification of uric acid stones with dual-energy

CT: diagnostic performance evaluation in patients. Abdom Imaging 2010;35(5):629–35.

35. Kulkarni NM, Eisner BH, Pinho DF, et al. Determination of renal stone composition in phantom and patients using single-source dual-energy computed tomography. J Comput Assist Tomogr 2013;37(1): 37–45.

36. Kalender WA, Klotz E, Suess C. Vertebral bone mineral analysis: an integrated approach with CT. Radiology 1987;164(2):419–23.

37. McCollough CH, Leng S, Yu L, et al. Dual- and multi-energy CT: principles, technical approaches, and clinical applications. Radiology 2015;276(3):637–53.

38. Leng S, Shiung M, Ai S, et al. Feasibility of discriminating uric acid from non-uric acid renal stones using consecutive spatially registered low- and high-energy scans obtained on a conventional CT scanner. AJR Am J Roentgenol 2015;204(1):92–7.

39. Chefd'hotel C, Hermosillo G, Faugeras O. Flows of diffeomorphisms for multimodal image registration. Proceedings IEEE International Symposium on Biomedical Imaging 2002;753–6.

40. Euler A, Parakh A, Falkowski AL, et al. Initial results of a single-source dual-energy computed tomography technique using a split-filter: assessment of image quality, radiation dose, and accuracy of dual-energy applications in an in vitro and in vivo study. Invest Radiol 2016;51(8):491–8.

41. Cai XR, Feng YZ, Qiu L, et al. Iodine distribution map in dual-energy computed tomography pulmonary artery imaging with rapid kVp switching for the diagnostic analysis and quantitative evaluation of acute pulmonary embolism. Acad Radiol 2015; 22(6):743–51.

42. Kiefer T, Diekhoff T, Hermann S, et al. Single source dual-energy computed tomography in the diagnosis of gout: diagnostic reliability in comparison to digital radiography and conventional computed tomography of the feet. Eur J Radiol 2016;85(10):1829–34.

43. Zhang D, Li X, Liu B. Objective characterization of GE discovery CT750 HD scanner: gemstone spectral imaging mode. Med Phys 2011;38(3):1178–88.

44. Petersilka M, Bruder H, Krauss B, et al. Technical principles of dual source CT. Eur J Radiol 2008; 68(3):362–8.

45. Hidas G, Eliahou R, Duvdevani M, et al. Determination of renal stone composition with dual-energy CT: in vivo analysis and comparison with x-ray diffraction. Radiology 2010;257(2):394–401.

46. Schlomka JP, Roessl E, Dorscheid R, et al. Experimental feasibility of multi-energy photon-counting K-edge imaging in pre-clinical computed tomography. Phys Med Biol 2008;53(15):4031–47.

47. Pourmorteza A, Symons R, Sandfort V, et al. Abdominal imaging with contrast-enhanced photon-counting CT: first human experience. Radiology 2016; 279(1):239–45.

48. Williamson JF, Li S, Devic S, et al. On two-parameter models of photon cross sections: application to dual-energy CT imaging. Med Phys 2006;33(11):4115–29.

49. Brooks RA. A quantitative theory of the Hounsfield unit and its application to dual energy scanning. J Comput Assist Tomogr 1977;1(4):487–93.

50. Brooks RA, Di Chiro G. Statistical limitations in x-ray reconstructive tomography. Med Phys 1976;3(4): 237–40.

51. Yu Z, Leng S, Kappler S, et al. Noise performance of low-dose CT: comparison between an energy integrating detector and a photon counting detector using a whole-body research photon counting CT scanner. J Med Imaging (Bellingham) 2016;3(4):043503.

52. McNitt-Gray MF. AAPM/RSNA physics tutorial for residents: topics in CT. Radiation dose in CT. Radiographics 2002;22(6):1541–53.

53. Yu L, Li H, Fletcher JG, et al. Automatic selection of tube potential for radiation dose reduction in CT: a general strategy. Med Phys 2010;37(1):234–43.

54. May MS, Brand M, Lell MM, et al. Radiation dose reduction in parasinus CT by spectral shaping. Neuroradiology 2017;59(2):169–76.

55. Kelcz F, Joseph PM, Hilal SK. Noise considerations in dual energy CT scanning. Med Phys 1979;6(5): 418–25.

56. Tawfik AM, Kerl JM, Razek AA, et al. Image quality and radiation dose of dual-energy CT of the head and neck compared with a standard 120-kVp acquisition. AJNR Am J Neuroradiol 2011;32(11):1994–9.

57. Krauss B, Grant KL, Schmidt BT, et al. The importance of spectral separation: an assessment of dual-energy spectral separation for quantitative ability and dose efficiency. Invest Radiol 2015;50(2):114–8.

58. Zatz LM. The effect of the kVp level on EMI values. Selective imaging of various materials with different kVp settings. Radiology 1976;119(3):683–8.

59. May MS, Bruegel J, Brand M, et al. Computed tomography of the head and neck region for tumor staging-comparison of dual-source, dual-energy and low-kilovolt, single-energy acquisitions. Invest Radiol 2017;52(9):522–8.

60. Faby S, Kuchenbecker S, Sawall S, et al. Performance of today's dual energy CT and future multi energy CT in virtual non-contrast imaging and in iodine quantification: a simulation study. Med Phys 2015; 42(7):4349–66.

61. McCollough CH, Bruesewitz MR, McNitt-Gray MF, et al. The phantom portion of the American College of Radiology (ACR) computed tomography (CT) accreditation program: practical tips, artifact examples, and pitfalls to avoid. Med Phys 2004;31(9): 2423–42.

62. Wiegert J, Engel KJ, Herrmann C. Impact of scattered radiation on spectral CT. In: Samei E; Hsieh J, editors. Proc. SPIE 7258, Medical Imaging 2009: Physics of Medical Imaging, 72583X; 2009. Available

at: http://spie.org/Publications/Proceedings/Paper/10.1117/12.813674.

63. Ananthakrishnan L, Rajiah P, Ahn R, et al. Spectral detector CT-derived virtual non-contrast images: comparison of attenuation values with unenhanced CT. Abdom Radiol (NY) 2017;42(3):702–9.

64. Toepker M, Moritz T, Krauss B, et al. Virtual non-contrast in second-generation, dual-energy computed tomography: reliability of attenuation values. Eur J Radiol 2012;81(3):e398–405.

65. Scholtz JE, Wichmann JL, Bennett DW, et al. Detecting intracranial hemorrhage using automatic tube current modulation with advanced modeled iterative reconstruction in unenhanced head single- and dual-energy dual-source CT. AJR Am J Roentgenol 2017;208(5):1089–96.

66. Rassouli N, Chalian H, Rajiah P, et al. Assessment of 70-keV virtual monoenergetic spectral images in abdominal CT imaging: a comparison study to conventional polychromatic 120-kVp images. Abdom Radiol (NY) 2017;42(10):2579–86.

67. Machida H, Fukui R, Tanaka I, et al. A method for selecting a protocol for routine body CT scan using Gemstone Spectral Imaging with or without adaptive statistical iterative reconstruction: phantom experiments. Jpn J Radiol 2014; 32(4):217–23.

68. Hyodo T, Yada N, Hori M, et al. Multimaterial decomposition algorithm for the quantification of liver fat content by using fast-kilovolt-peak switching dual-energy CT: clinical evaluation. Radiology 2017; 283(1):108–18.

69. De Cecco CN, Darnell A, Macías N, et al. Virtual unenhanced images of the abdomen with second-generation dual-source dual-energy computed tomography: image quality and liver lesion detection. Invest Radiol 2013;48(1):1–9.

70. Pache G, Krauss B, Strohm P, et al. Dual-energy CT virtual noncalcium technique: detecting posttraumatic bone marrow lesions–feasibility study. Radiology 2010;256(2):617–24.

71. Kellock TT, Nicolaou S, Kim SSY, et al. Detection of bone marrow edema in nondisplaced hip fractures: utility of a virtual noncalcium dual-energy CT application. Radiology 2017;284(3):798–805.

72. Petritsch B, Kosmala A, Weng AM, et al. Vertebral compression fractures: third-generation dual-energy CT for detection of bone marrow edema at visual and quantitative analyses. Radiology 2017;284(1):161–8.

73. Andreini D, Pontone G, Mushtaq S, et al. Diagnostic accuracy of rapid kilovolt peak-switching dual-energy CT coronary angiography in patients with a high calcium score. JACC Cardiovasc Imaging 2015;8(6):746–8.

Dual-Energy Computed Tomography
Image Acquisition, Processing, and Workflow

Alec J. Megibow, MD, MPH[a],*,
Avinash Kambadakone, MD, DNB, FRCR[b],
Lakshmi Ananthakrishnan, MD[c]

KEYWORDS

- Dual energy CT • Dual energy CT methods • Dual energy workflow
- Clinical integration of dual energy CT

KEY POINTS

- The basic image acquisition method of 3 major dual energy computed tomography acquisition platforms is described.
- How dual energy computed tomography data is integrated from workstation to clinical reading is presented.
- Presentation modes of various dual energy computed tomography reconstructions applicable to abdominal imaging are discussed.

INTRODUCTION

Dual energy computed tomography (DECT) is an acquisition method where images are obtained at 2 different energies. The potential benefits of DECT over single energy acquisitions were envisioned by Hounsfield in his original article describing CT systems. Hounsfield understood that by acquiring images at 2 different energies, one could "use the machine for determining the atomic number of the material within the slice."[1] Considerable technical issues had to be overcome before Hounsfield's 1973 vision was realized in the first clinical scanner introduced in 2006.[2] Since that time, all of the major CT manufacturers have introduced dual energy systems, each with a different design, but all capable of acquiring and processing images at 2 different energy spectra. These include dual source dual energy systems (DSDECT) from Siemens Medical Systems (Forcheim, Germany), single source rapid kV switching systems (rsDECT) from General Electric Medical Systems (Milwaukee, WI), dual layer spectral detector CT (SDCT) from Philips Medical Systems (Einthoven, the Netherlands; Fig. 1). Siemens offers 2 single source DECT options as well, including a shuttle acquisition where patients are scanned with 1 kV in cephalocaudad direction and immediately rescanned at a second kV in the caudad-cephalad direction, and more recently, a split gold/tin filter placed between the x-ray source and the patient resulting in a single beam with

Disclosure Statement: Consultant, Bracco Diagnostics Inc (A.J. Megibow).
[a] Department of Radiology, NYU-Langone Medical Center, 550 First Avenue, Room HCC 232, New York, NY 10016, USA; [b] Department of Radiology, Harvard Medical School, Massachusetts General Hospital, 55 Fruit Street, White 270, Boston, MA 02114, USA; [c] Department of Radiology, University of Texas Southwestern Medical Center, 5323 Harry Hines Boulevard, Dallas, TX 75390-8827, USA
* Corresponding author.
E-mail address: alec.megibow@nyumc.org

Radiol Clin N Am 56 (2018) 507–520
https://doi.org/10.1016/j.rcl.2018.03.001

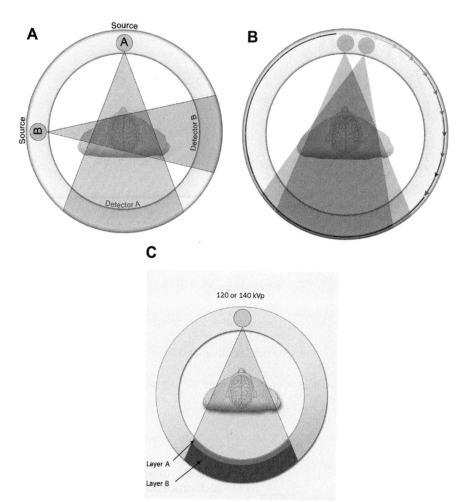

Fig. 1. (*A*) Dual source dual energy computed tomography (DSDECT): 2 tubes offset at 95° expose 2 separate detectors. The "A" tube and detector has a field of view equivalent to a single source CT scanner. The "B" tube and detector has a 35-cm field of view. Dual energy information is only available in that portion of the anatomy traversed by both beams. (*B*) Rapid kV switching DECT (rsDECT): A single tube rotates around the patient rapidly changing kV from 140 to 80 kV as indicated by the "red state" (high kV) and "blue state" (low kV) exposing a single detector. There is no limitation to the dual energy calculations within the entire field of view. (*C*) Spectral DECT (SDCT). A single tube exposes the patient at either 120 or 140 kVp. Spectral separation occurs at the detector level where the yttrium based inner layer A separates low energy photons allowing the high-energy photons to interact with the gadolinium oxysulfide based outer layer B, which absorbs the high-energy photons.

spectral separation. Currently, there is limited clinical experience with the single source rapid switching DECT based on gantry rotation from Toshiba Medical Systems (Otawara, Japan).

Although the novelty and "potential" of DECT excites radiologists anxious to offer this technology to patients, many purchased systems, regardless of manufacturer, are underused. The reasons for this are difficult to explain, although the most frequently heard resistance from radiologists is related to limited specific indications for dual energy imaging, perceived radiation dose penalty, time pressures in busy practices, multiplicity of images requiring increased reading time per case,

lack of "trust" of dual energy data, particularly regarding Hounsfield unit determination, and, not insignificantly, no available billing codes that recognize the extra work radiologists perform when interpreting these studies.

Those of us who have experience with DECT can attest to the tremendous usefulness of this technology in day-to-day radiology practice; for wider clinical dissemination, an understanding of how the images are acquired and the workflow(s) needed to present these dual energy images to the radiologist becomes imperative. Herein, we attempt to provide detailed descriptions of how images are acquired and processed in DSDECT, rsDECT, and SDCT systems and to illustrate how these images are integrated into clinical radiology practice. The subsequent articles in this edition of the Clinics will detail the many applications of DECT in body imaging.

DUAL SOURCE DUAL ENERGY COMPUTED TOMOGRAPHY
Image Acquisition and Reconstruction

DSDECT scanners acquire images from 2 separate tubes offset by 95°. The high kV tube operates at a fixed kVp of either 140 or 150 depending on the model of scanner and has a full field of view equivalent to a single source conventional CT scanner. The low kV tube can operate at variable kVp from 70 to 100; the kV setting for a particular examination depends on patient size. This tube has a field of view limited to 35 cm (see **Fig. 1A**). Experienced technologists can position larger patients such that the relevant anatomy is within the reconstruction circle. In our practice, we rely on technologist judgment to determine if a given patient can be scanned in dual energy mode. In our practice, we routinely scan using 150/80 kVp because this setting gives excellent spectral separation with minimal noise. For pediatric patients, we use 150/70 kVp.

For thoracic and abdominal imaging, the images are acquired at a pitch of 0.6. We routinely use a 0.6 mm detector width, resulting in isotropic voxels measuring 0.65 mm. Separate image data from the high kV and low kV tubes are reconstructed and automatically sent to a thin client workstation (SyngoVia VB20, Siemens Medical Solutions, Malvern PA). DECT processing engines are embedded in the workstation that immediately begin processing these 2 image streams into a linear blended set of images and a variety of other data displays that the user can choose based on the type of scan and clinical needs. The linear blended images are based on a preset user preference for final image appearance that simulates a CT image as if acquired by a single source scanner. In our department, we choose a 50%/50% high/low kV blending when we scan with 150 kVp and a 60%/40% high/low kV blending when scanning with a 140 kVp system. These blended images are simultaneously sent to the picture archiving and communication system (PACS) as 4 mm axial and 3 mm coronal sections (**Fig. 2**) provides an overview of this workflow.

DUAL ENERGY WORKFLOW

Currently, we have 2 Somatom FORCE DSDECT (Siemens Medical Solutions) scanners; one functions as the sole CT scanner in our emergency department, the other is one of 2 scanners in our outpatient area. We acquire dual energy data as

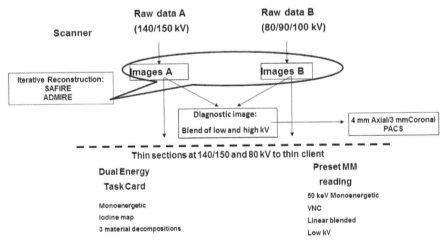

Fig. 2. Dual source dual energy computed tomography (DSDECT) workflow. Raw data from each tube are separately reconstructed at scanner into 2 image bins (images A and B). Dual energy–specific iterative reconstructions are applied to both datasets during the reconstruction process. The bins are automatically blended in terms of percentage of kV contribution into a diagnostic image and user specified slice thicknesses are sent to the picture archiving and communication system (PACS). The interpreting radiologist will frequently only view these images. Simultaneously, 2 thin section bins are sent to the thin client. Here they are "postprocessed" in the background. Postprocessing choices depend on the type of scan and the clinical indication. These images can be viewed on a dual energy card where a variety of operations such as user-varied monoenergetic reconstructions, iodine maps, or advanced 3 material decompositions can be created, or on an "multimodality reading card" where preset reconstructions including 50 keV monoenergetic, virtual noncontrast (VNC), linear blended and low kV images are displayed.

the primary acquisition mode for all patients who are examined on those particular scanners. In the outpatient area, we have the ability to apply protocols to scheduled patients up to 5 weeks in advance of their appointment. Therefore, if there is a particular case that specifically requires dual energy scanning, we can prospectively assign that patient to the appropriate machine.

Our workflow is based on the principle that the dual energy data is available in one of the following ways: (a) as a problem solving tool, such as determining presence of enhancement or a noncontrast Hounsfield unit value; (b) for enhanced iodine conspicuity, such as for either contrast media volume reduction or visualizing small arteries such as in evaluation of perforator arteries; (c) to eliminate acquisitions with attendant decrease in overall radiation dose; and (d) iodine quantification for the assessment of tumor or inflammatory neovascularity. Implicit is the fact that, in many cases, the dual energy data may not even be looked at.[3] Because the blended images presented to the radiologist on the PACS system have all of the properties of a standard CT image, radiologists can window, obtain Hounsfield unit readings, measure diameters as if reading conventionally acquired CT images. We do not send all of the dual energy images to PACS; our radiologists therefore do not feel obligated to look at images that may have limited if any diagnostic value in a particular case.

Simultaneous to the image transfer to PACS, the scanner also sends 0.6 mm slices from both the 150 kV and the low kV acquisitions to the thin client workstation. Once these images are received on the workstation, they are processed into preset dual energy–related image sets. Correct processing of dual energy data requires appropriate mapping rules to be created. Images from the scanner are tagged with a prefix "#pp"; when the workstation sees this on a set of images, it will know how to process the case. This mapping is set up at the time of scanner installation and embedded into examination protocols. For a typical abdominal–pelvic examination, this setting results in approximately 900 images per tube or a total of 1800 images. Slices are reconstructed at a rate of 20 images per second, so the entire reconstruction task is 1.5 minutes. Background processing of these images into DECT data depends on the number of requested image types.

The dual energy application on the thin client workstation is displays images in 2 separate areas; a "dual energy (DE) card" and a "multimodality (MM) reading card." Axial, sagittal, and coronal 0.6 mm sections are displayed on a 4:1 display on the DE card along with a "place holder." Based on the application profile of the examination (eg, abdomen with contrast vs abdomen without contrast), a suite of up to 4 operations can be chosen, each of which is a specified 3-material decomposition[4] appropriate for the native acquisition. Specifically, for a contrast enhanced study, we can create monoenergetic images at any KeV (although our default level is 50 KeV), "liver VNC (virtual noncontrast)" images specifically designed for hepatic imaging, "virtual unenhanced" (VUE) images with similar functionality for all areas outside the liver, and "body bone removal" that uses dual energy imaging to remove the bones. We use the liver VNC and VUE images to create an iodine map from which a dual energy region of interest circle can automatically display contrast enhancement levels and iodine "density" (**Fig. 3**A). For unenhanced studies, a "kidney stone" option is available that, when selected, will provide the stone diameter, volume Hounsfield unit level, and dual energy ratio.

We have configured the MM reading card to display a routinely created "VNC" dataset and a 50 KeV monoenergetic dataset. These image sets are immediately available as a linked 4:1 display (**Fig. 3**B). We also display the linear blended mixed image and images from the low KeV tube. The fully processed images displayed on the MM reading card retain Hounsfield unit values that can be read on the PACS system. It is important to remember that Hounsfield unit readings should only be recorded on the linear blended mixed images or the VNC. All of the displays are of 0.6 mm slices, which allows the creation of multiplanar reformatted, maximum intensity projection, and volume rendered images independent from any of the reconstructions.

Image Networking and Archiving

The routine use of dual energy acquisition creates a challenge for image management. A single dual energy acquisition will produce 3 times the number of images (high kV, low kV, and blended) one would create from a single energy study. Because the scanner acquires at minimal detector width, the number of images per case can rapidly accumulate. To avoid burdening our PACS system, the scanner only sends 4 mm axial and 3 mm coronal images to the PACS. All of the thin slices are sent to the thin client. Images from the thin client are not routinely archived onto PACS. We "delete protect" cases of particular interest or teaching value. Recently, our department purchased server space that accepts the high and low kV acquisitions for long-term storage. We do not send the various postprocessed images to this site. If a

A

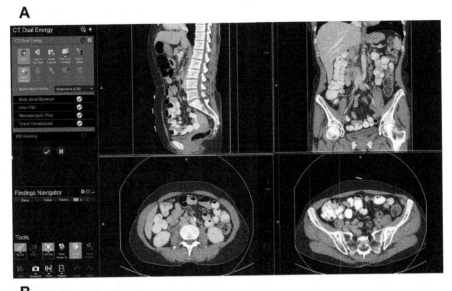

B

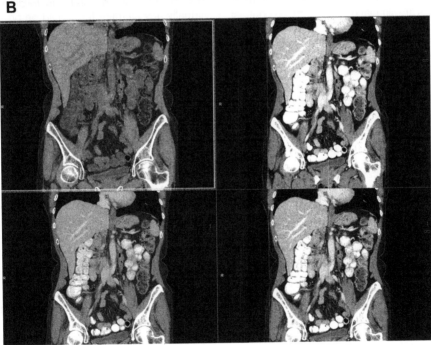

Fig. 3. (*A*) Dual source dual energy computed tomography (DSDECT) dual energy display. Blended images are available on the dual energy card, a list of possible viewing modes appears on the left. (*B*) DSDECT multimodality reading card. Preprocessed thin section images include (*top*) virtual noncontrast, 50 keV monoenergetic and (*bottom*) linear blended and low kV image. All of these images are readily available for 3-dimensional viewing and display. Moving from the dual energy card to the multimodality reading card is a single mouse click.

case is retrieved, it needs to be re-reconstructed from the native datasets.

USEFULNESS OF DUAL ENERGY DATA

The many applications of DECT are highlighted elsewhere in this issue. However, it is useful to address the accuracy of Hounsfield unit values determined from VNC images derived from a DSDECT. Published reports show that, in 91% of patients, the true noncontrast (TNC) and VNC Hounsfield unit values are within 15 Hounsfield units[5] and could be reliable in documenting renal cysts and incidental adrenal masses.[6,7] In our own practice, we are comfortable in eliminating TNC acquisitions for CT urograms, aortic endograft studies,[8] gastrointestinal bleeding evaluation,[9] and oncologic imaging.[10] We find the iodine maps are most useful for assessing the presence or absence of enhancement because regions of iodine uptake are more easily detected against in a predominantly cystic, necrotic or treated[11] lesion.

The iodine density in milligrams per milliliter of iodine can also be determined from the iodine map. DSDECT scanners have been shown to be accurate in determining the concentration of iodine in solutions.[12,13] This value can be thought of as a surrogate measure of the neovascularity and may be useful in monitoring antiangiogenic[12] or antiinflammatory therapies. Some investigators have proposed that iodine density as a surrogate measure or perfusion.[14,15]

The use of virtual monochromatic (VMC) images has been shown to reduce variability in CT numbers. These images are simulations of the image contrast that might be seen had the image been created by a beam of a single energy.[16] Aside from the increased contrast-to-noise ratio (CNR) inherent in these images, CT numbers are also more stable.[17,18] This knowledge is useful in attempting to determine true enhancement from pseudoenhancement,[19] thereby avoiding misdiagnosis.

RADIATION DOSE CONSIDERATIONS

Overall patient dose can be decreased by eliminating acquisitions, substituting VNC images for a TNC acquisition. Although one might first think that a system using 2 separate tubes would double the radiation to the patient, this is not the case. The total dose delivered in a single rotation of a single energy scan is *shared* between the 2 tubes, resulting in dose-neutral acquisitions. Noise reduction iterative reconstruction methods are routinely applied in the reconstruction phase. A special reconstruction "Q" kernel has been developed specifically for dual energy data. Studies have documented no degradation in image quality when DSDECT datasets are compared with single energy datasets in unmatched[20] or matched[21] patient populations.

RAPID kV SWITCHING DUAL ENERGY COMPUTED TOMOGRAPHY
Image Acquisition

The single source or rapid kVp switching DECT (rsDECT) scanner (Discovery CT 750 HD; GE Healthcare) has a single x-ray tube source capable of rapidly switching between low- and high-energy settings (80 and 140 kVp) and a single detector layer, which enables swift sampling of the

alternating energy data to permit dual energy scanning[3,22] (see **Fig. 1**B). The rapid kVp switching technology permits a full field of effective dual energy scanning (50 cm) while allowing optimal temporal registration between the high- and low-energy datasets.[3,23,24] To compensate for the lack of automatic tube current modulation and higher tube output with the 140 kVp acquisition, the 80/140 kVp exposure time ratio is maintained at 65%/35%, thereby maximizing the CNR.[23]

As opposed to DSDECT systems, raw dual energy data for material analysis occurs before reconstruction of images from the high and low energy sinograms (ie, in data domain or projection space decomposition).[24,25] Projection space decomposition has the benefits of greater flexibility in the types of materials that can be used for decompositions and preprocessing correction of data to minimize beam hardening artifacts.[24,25] This flexibility allows users to easily interrogate virtually any element that could be present within a region of interest as opposed to DSDECT systems requiring the manufacturer to create a custom 3-material decomposition.

The rsDECT scanners in our practice serve both inpatients and outpatients and the scheduling of patients on these scanners is performed based on availability through a centralized scheduling service. Our rsDECT workflow has been designed to be technologist centric. We ask the CT technologists to play an integral role in patient selection, image acquisition, data processing, and image relay to the PACS for interpretation and diagnosis. For this reason, it is very important to have expert CT technologists who understand the local image network, departmental expectations of image quality, and its workflow challenges. The technologist determines if a patient can be appropriately imaged with DECT based on body habitus and examination protocols. Generally, patients weighing more than 260 pounds (118 kg) are not selected for DE scanning, owing to image quality degradation arising from increased image noise and photon starvation. There may be insufficient mA available to maintain photon flux particularly from the low energy acquisition, which is limited to 80 kV.[3]

To maximize efficiency and simplify workflow, we perform rsDECT scanning based on specific examination protocols rather than clinical indications, for example, a multiphasic liver or renal mass protocol. This approach automates the image acquisition process and renders the implementation of DECT easier in a busy CT practice.[26] Specific protocols are assigned to the CT examination using an electronic protocoling system, for example, a multiphasic pancreatic protocol DECT is assigned for a patient with a suspected pancreatic mass.[3,26] The rsDECT scanner has the most updated CT protocols (both single energy and dual energy) with appropriate technical parameters for the technologist to choose from.[3,26] For example, a patient with alcoholic cirrhosis (weighing 180 lbs) scheduled on a DECT scanner for surveillance of the liver the technologist selects the multiphasic liver mass DECT protocol from the scanner. In contrast, if the same patient weighed 280 lbs the technologist selects a multiphasic single energy CT (SECT) liver mass protocol for hepatic imaging on the rsDECT scanner.

Reconstruction

After image acquisition, reconstruction of raw dual energy data on the rsDECT scanner is automated. Automatic postprocessing allows the technologist to continue with other tasks, such as removing the intravenous line, walking the patient out of the room, and setting up the room for next patient. These automated reconstruction processes take approximately 5 minutes to complete. This delay does not interfere with patient flow, because the processing of an initial patient can proceed while a subsequent patient is being scanned. However, the PACS and/or the workstation cannot receive images until all processing has been completed. The creation of preset protocols with detailed instructions on reconstruction of various image datasets makes the technologist's job easier and streamlines workflow. The image datasets generated on the scanner should be chosen to maximize material-specific information unique to DECT as well as providing high-quality diagnostic images for patient diagnosis. The number and type of image datasets for each specific protocol has been already predetermined at the time of protocol creation. Image presets should be optimized such that the minimum numbers of images essential for diagnostic interpretation are generated while reducing scanner processing time, limiting the burden on PACS storage space and decreasing radiologist interpretation time.[26]

On the rsDECT scanner, the acquired 140 and 80 kVp projections are reconstructed in the projection space to generate multiple image datasets based on type of protocol.[3,24] For example, for a routine cancer follow-up portal venous phase abdomen–pelvis CT protocol, we generate the following images: (a) axial 5 mm thick 140 kVp quality control (QC) images, (b) axial 5 mm thick 65 keV VMC images, (c) axial 5 mm thick material density–water images, (d) axial 5 mm thick material density–iodine images, and (e) coronal/sagittal images (3 mm). To begin with, there is immediate creation of 140 kVp QC images (5 mm thickness) on the scanner console

that allow the technologists to verify the images for adequacy of anatomic coverage and contrast media opacification. Unlike DSDECT, 80 kVp images are not routinely created to reduce scanner processing time. **Fig. 4** provides an overview of the workflow.

Two standard image datasets, with appropriate calibration, are automatically generated on the scanner, and include (a) virtual monoenergetic (VMC) images at a preselected energy level (keV) and (b) material density pair images.[24] Although VMC images can be obtained at any desired energy level (40–140 keV), we usually process 1 set of VMC images per phase of acquisition. For intravenous contrast-enhanced CT scans of the abdomen and pelvis, VMC images at photon energy level of 60 to 77 keV are reported to have an optimal peak CNR.[24,26] In our practice, the arterial phase VMC images are generally reconstructed at 50 keV (low energy, 2.5 mm slice thickness) and portal venous phase images are reconstructed at 65 keV (medium energy, 5 mm slice thickness). The 50 keV images significantly enhance the iodine content based on enhanced photoelectric-like contribution to the image. The 65 keV images generated resemble a single energy 120 kVp SECT study, but with higher tissue and intravascular CNR. Additionally, thin section (0.625–1.250 mm) axial VMC images are also reconstructed to enable creation of coronal and sagittal reformatted images (3 mm thickness). Higher keV, VMC images (ie, at 120 and 140 keV) can be created for metal artifact reduction.

The 2-material decomposition algorithm used in rsDECT creates material density pair images such as iodine–water, fat–iodine, and calcium–iodine. In our practice, we routinely create a pair of iodine–water images (5 mm slice thickness), which includes (a) material density iodine image depicting iodine distribution within the tissues and (b) water density image, which is similar to a true unenhanced image. Thin section images from these images are available only on the workstation (**Fig. 5**).

All the image datasets created on the scanner are sent to PACS for radiologist interpretation except the thin section VMC images, which are used only for the creation of multiplanar reformations. The rsDECT scanner allows image acquisition with isotropic voxels (0.625 mm) that has complete 3-dimensional capability once the final images are reconstructed. A standalone dedicated workstation is located in the CT scanner area, which enables additional postprocessing of the DECT datasets, such as additional VMC images of varying KeV levels, additional basis pair images, spectral curve, and effective z

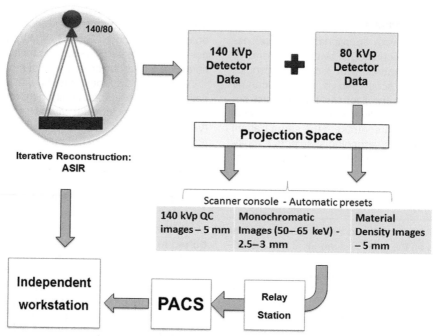

Fig. 4. Rapid switching dual energy computed tomography (rsDECT) workflow. Dual energy scanning (140/80 kVp) is performed using rapid kVp switching and application of ASIR. The acquired 140 and 80 kVp detector are reconstructed in the projection space on the scanner console automatically to generate the preset image datasets (140 kVp quality control, virtual monochromatic, and material density images). The coronal and sagittal reformatted images are generated from the virtual monochromatic images on the scanner by the technologist. The images are then routed to the relay station before transmission to the PACS. For additional postprocessing, the images can be transmitted to an independent workstation either from PACS or directly from the scanner. ASIR, adaptive statistical iterative reconstruction; PACS, picture archiving and communication system.

maps, and these are used for research purposes, for example, the creation of varying KeV levels to optimize hyperenhancing liver lesion detection. DECT images can either be relayed to this workstation directly from the scanner or retrieved from PACS. We do not use a thin client server on our PACS workstation for additional postprocessing during routine interpretation.

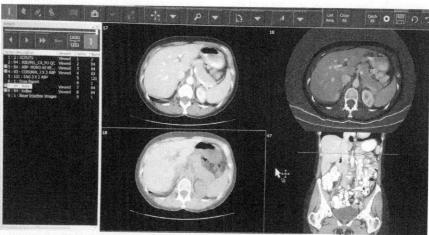

Fig. 5. Picture archiving and communication system (PACS) display of rapid switching dual energy computed tomography (rsDECT) data. Typical contrast-enhanced DECT dataset from a cancer follow-up abdomen/pelvis CT scan. The series tab along the left side of the display shows the various DECT series sent to PACS for radiologist interpretation. The 4 image datasets displayed include (*top left*) a 5-mm axial 65 keV monochromatic image series, (*top right*) a 5-mm axial material density iodine image, (*bottom left*) a 5-mm axial material density water image, and (*bottom right*) a 3-mm coronal reformatted image.

The processing time for DECT image datasets on the scanner console is slightly longer than a comparable SECT study owing to the increased number of image series; examination time increases as more imaging phases are added. For example, a single portal venous phase abdominal DECT scan generates 1200 to 1500 images, whereas a similar SECT protocol generates 350 to 550 images. The estimated examination time for a routine single phase abdomen pelvis DECT scan from the time of starting of scan acquisition to the images being available in PACS is about 15 to 20 minutes, whereas a similar SECT scan takes 10 to 15 minutes.

Workflow

For interpretation, the radiologists review all the DECT image datasets archived into the PACS. Additional postprocessing either using a thin client server or on the separate workstation is not routinely required and is not feasible considering our busy practice. Although the approach for interpreting a DECT scan varies between radiologists, most readers review images in the following order: 140 kVp QC, VMC, material density iodine, VUE, and coronal/sagittal reformatted images. The VMC images are less affected by beam hardening artifacts and provide more stable Hounsfield unit values than SECT images that are less susceptible to pseudoenhancement.[17,19,27] There are reported variations in the mean attenuation values of 5 to 15 Hounsfield units among different organs between true unenhanced and VUE images.[27–29] On rsDECT, region of interest evaluation of VUE images does not provide Hounsfield unit values, which limits their usefulness for quantitative evaluation. Therefore, we often rely on subjective evaluation of lesions on VUE to determine precontrast density.[28,29]

Quantitative estimation of iodine distribution in tissues can be performed using regions of interest that provide iodine concentration in milligrams per milliliter. The reported iodine density threshold for detection of enhancement in renal lesions is between 1.28 and 2.00 mgI/mL.[23,30,31] We often rely on subjective assessment to determine enhancement during the review of iodine images. Color overlay iodine maps and graphical spectral attenuation curves allow improved detection of enhancement however they are of limited practical value in our practice because they need to be created on the standalone workstation.

Indications

The proven benefits of DECT in the abdomen include characterization of focal liver and pancreatic lesions, determination of urinary stone composition, vascular imaging, and renal mass characterization.[30] The ability to use lower KeV VMC allows decreases in the iodinated contrast dose by approximately 30% in all patients, especially those with borderline renal function.

DE acquisitions are variably used based on clinical indications. For most patients, referred for CT for abdominal pain evaluation or a routine cancer follow-up study, DECT is performed in the single portal venous phase.[10]

For multiphasic liver CT studies, we perform DECT in the arterial phase because lower energy VMC datasets provide improved conspicuity of hypervascular tumors, such as hepatocellular carcinoma.[10] In addition, DECT images enable improved differentiation of bland from tumor thrombus and posttreatment assessment after locoregional therapies such as ablation and transarterial chemoembolization.[10,11,32,33] Conversely, multiphasic pancreatic protocol CT includes DE scanning in both the arterial/pancreatic portal venous phases, improving pancreatic mass detection and liver lesion detection. We do not acquire TNC images because VUE images usually are sufficient.[26] For evaluation of mesenteric/bowel ischemia and gastrointestinal bleeding source, we use DE acquisition in the arterial phase and single energy acquisition for the portal venous/delayed phase. The low energy VMC and iodine images allow improved detection of detection of source of bleeding and bowel wall enhancement for bowel ischemia.

For renal mass protocol CT and CT urography, we acquire a TNC SECT examinations followed by a DECT nephrographic phase examination. The delayed excretory phase acquisition during a CT urography study is performed in the single energy mode. VUE images potentially could replace true unenhanced acquisitions reducing radiation dose in genitourinary CT studies currently performed with and without contrast. However, current quantitative limitations of VUE images pertaining to accurate Hounsfield unit values arising when unenhanced portion is acquired from DECT data has limited our adaptation.[26] In patients undergoing stone protocol CT scans, we initially perform a SECT for the abdomen and pelvis followed by a targeted DE acquisition in the region of stone to allow assessment of stone composition and limit radiation dose.[34,35]

RADIATION DOSE CONSIDERATIONS

For a particular examination protocol, the radiation dose associated with rsDECT is comparable with or lower than with SECT.[36,37] Newer scanners with application of iterative reconstruction techniques enable a reduction in the noise in rsDECT scans with the ability to use a lower dose. DECT also enables dose reduction associated with CT scans by eliminating individual phases in multiphasic examinations, reducing the number of additional CT studies.[24]

SPECTRAL DETECTOR COMPUTED TOMOGRAPHY
Image Acquisition

The dual layer SDCT system uses a single x-ray beam source that emits a typical polychromatic x-ray beam, similar to that used in conventional SECT. As opposed to DSDECT and rsDECT, spectral separation occurs at the detector level, after the x-ray beam has interacted with the patient[38,39] (see Fig. 1C). The superficial layer of the detector (inner layer closest to the patient) is composed of yttrium, and absorbs the lower energy photons while allowing the higher energy photons to pass through to the deeper detector layer. The deeper detector layer is made of gadolinium oxysulfide and has a high rate of absorption for these higher energy photons. This differential absorption of low and high energy photons by the dual layer detector is greatest at beam energies of 120 and 140 kVp; thus, although conventional CT images may be obtained while operating the x-ray tube source at lower tube potentials of 80 or 100 kVp, spectral reconstructions are available only when imaging is performed at 120 or 140 kVp. Because spectral separation is performed after the polychromatic x-ray beam has passed through the patient, spectral data on this scanner are spatially coregistered.

The image acquisition at the x-ray source level is performed in a similar manner as single energy scanners from the same manufacturer. Slice thickness, pitch, and other scan parameters may be determined by the user. During image acquisition, traditional dose saving methods such as tube current modulation in the x, y, and z axes and iterative reconstruction methods (iDose and iMR, Philips Healthcare) are available. There are 64 detector rows with individual detector element width of 0.625 mm; total detector width is 4 cm. In our clinical experience to date, the radiation dose delivered with this system is equivalent to conventional scanners. However, further studies are needed for confirmation for different anatomic locations.

Image Reconstruction

The information from the 2 layers of the detector may be displayed in 2 different methods. The first is the "conventional" reconstruction. This is a weighted combination of the data from each detector layer, creating an image that most closely resembles a 120 or 140 kVp image from a single energy scanner. This conventional image is conceptually similar to the "linear blended" image created on the dual source system.

The second method of image reconstruction is creation of a "spectral base image" (SBI) series at the scanner console. The low and high energy sinograms from each detector layer are converted into photoelectric and Compton sinograms, which are then combined into the SBI series. Because the spectral data are coregistered, this reconstruction process is performed in the projection space, before image reconstruction. This methodology allows for theoretically improved beam hardening correction.[39] From this SBI series, any spectral reconstruction may be created retrospectively on demand by the user, either in the thin client (Intellispace Portal, Philips Healthcare) or by using the "on the fly" analysis tool (Magic Glass, Philips Healthcare), described elsewhere in this article. Alternatively, if a single reconstruction is desired for every case (eg, 50 KeV monoenergetic image), this image may be prospectively created at the scanner console and sent to the PACS. This process may be built into the protocol on the scanner, automating the process and eliminating any extra steps for the technologist. Fig. 6 provides an overview of the workflow. In the current version of the software, each SBI series takes approximately 3 to 5 minutes to create, but the vendor is that actively working to significantly reduce the reconstruction time.

Types of spectral reconstructions available on the SDCT platform are similar to those available on DSDECT or ssDECT platforms, and include virtual monoenergetic images, VNC images, and iodine quantification (iodine-no-water) reconstructions. Attenuation measurements on VNC images are displayed in Hounsfield units. One study comparing Hounsfield units between VNC and TNC images on the SDCT platform in multiple structures in the abdomen found that attenuation was within 10 Hounsfield units in most structures, with the exception of fat.[38] Attenuation in fat was slightly overestimated on VNC images compared with TNC images, a phenomenon seen on other platforms as well.[40] Iodine-no-water reconstructions display iodine concentration in milligrams per milliliter. Phantom studies have shown good fidelity between measured and actual iodine concentration. In addition, several segmentation reconstructions are available, including iodine density images (segmenting out calcium), uric acid removed (segmenting out uric acid), and uric acid (segmenting out calcium) reconstructions.

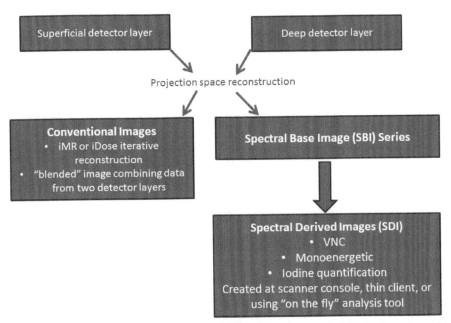

Fig. 6. Spectral dual energy computed tomography workflow. Data from each detector layer is combined in the projection space, and may be reconstructed to create 2 different datasets: (1) conventional images, and (2) spectral base images, which can then be used to create any desired spectral reconstruction (termed spectral-derived image) on demand. VNC, virtual noncontrast.

Image Storage and Viewing

The SBI series must be created at the scanner console and is approximately 3 to 4 times the size of the conventional dataset. Because any spectral reconstruction may be rapidly created from this series, we send the SBI series for every case to the thin client for temporary viewing and storage, but also choose to permanently store the SBI series on the PACS in all cases so we may access the spectral data in the future if desired.

There are 3 different options for viewing spectral data: any spectral reconstruction on PACS and SBI reconstructions in a thin client environment without or with Magic Glass on the fly. PACS viewing of spectral reconstructions are familiar to radiologists, but suffer minor limitations. Attenuation measurements may be obtained in PACS itself on reconstructions that provide attenuation (ie, VNC and virtual monoenergetic images); however, iodine quantification measurements cannot be made in PACS, as with DSDECT systems. The SBI series allows viewing any spectral reconstruction on demand. The SBI series may be opened in the thin client, and any spectral reconstruction may be created and viewed for the entire CT dataset within a few seconds. In our practice, the thin client may be accessed from any PACS station, and thus a separate spectral workstation is not needed. Last, the Magic Glass may be launched directly in the PACS, which allows quick access to the spectral data without opening the thin client. This analysis tool allows for viewing of 2 different reconstructions; the user may choose which reconstructions are displayed. The PACS Magic Glass has most of the functionality that is available in the thin client, including the ability to obtain measurements; however, it is restricted to a limited field of view within the image. In our practice, we find that the majority of analysis (including obtaining measurements) may be performed in this PACS Magic Glass tool without opening up the thin client. The Magic Glass is also available for use in the thin client; here, 4 different reconstructions may be viewed for a single selected field of view. In both the PACS and thin client Magic Glass, the field of view may be resized and moved to allow interrogation of lesions of different sizes and location. Measurements obtained in the PACS or thin client Magic Glass tool may be captured and sent to PACS (**Fig. 7**).

WHEN TO USE DUAL ENERGY COMPUTED TOMOGRAPHY

Once a patient is on the SDCT scanner, there is no need to prospectively decide which phase of

A

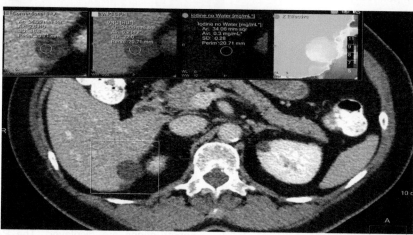

B

Fig. 7. (*A*) Spectral detector computed tomography image types. Typical reconstructions include iodine maps that can be used for iodine quantification and monoenergetic displays at user selected keV, 70 in this example, that can accentuate iodine signal. (*B*) Use of Magic Glass. The Magic Glass "on the fly" analysis tool launched in thin client. This tool is useful for interrogation of specific lesions. The green box (indicating the field of view) may be moved or adjusted for size. Four view boxes are available in the thin client, and displayed spectral reconstructions may be changed by the user. Measurements may be taken directly in Magic Glass.

imaging to use dual energy mode: because spectral separation is performed retrospectively, the spectral data are available on demand for any scan performed at 120 or 140 kVp. In a busy clinical practice, the radiologist may choose to triage certain cases to this scanner where the spectral data may be of benefit. Potential candidates for SDCT include oncologic and vascular cases for improved iodine conspicuity, CT urograms for elimination of a TNC phase and radiation dose reduction, and emergency room cases for incidentaloma characterization. At the authors' institution, our scanner is located in an inpatient/emergency room setting. Although the SDCT scanner is preferentially used if available, priority is given to contrast-enhanced abdominal examinations (for incidentaloma characterization and lesion detection capabilities), and CT angiograms of the aorta, pulmonary arteries, and head and neck.

An important point to consider is reconstruction times: it currently takes approximately 3 to 5 minutes to reconstruct the SBI series at the scanner, although the reconstruction may occur in the background on the scanner while the technologist moves on to the next patient. As stated, the vendor will correct the reconstruction times in the near future.

Because the first commercially available SDCT scanner in the United States was installed in 2016, there are few published data to date regarding its use for clinical applications. As with other DECT methods, SDCT can be used to improve lesion/iodine conspicuity, decreasing beam hardening artifacts, and decrease contrast load for CT angiography. Clinical applications in abdominal and pelvic imaging include the use of low virtual monoenergetic imaging to improve organ CNR and decrease noise compared with conventional imaging in the abdomen.[41] High virtual monoenergetic (74–150 KeV) images in patients with hip prostheses showed improved CNR.[42] For abdominal CT angiograms, the use of lower KeV images may allow creation of a "virtual arterial phase," potentially decreasing the number of phases needed to detect an endoleak after stent graft placement. Preliminary clinical experience shows usefulness of SDCT reconstructions in improving image quality in CT pulmonary angiograms with a suboptimal contrast bolus, as well as detecting perfusion defects.[43] Thus far, no studies have been performed assessing the impact of patient size on image quality on the SDCT platform. In these authors' experience, a particular strength of the SDCT platform is in characterizing incidental lesions using the Magic Glass on-the-fly analysis tool owing to the ease of retrospective access to multiple types of reconstructions.

REFERENCES

1. Hounsfield GN. Computerized transverse axial scanning (tomography). 1. Description of system. Br J Radiol 1973;46(552):1016–22.

2. Flohr TG, McCollough CH, Bruder H, et al. First performance evaluation of a dual-source CT (DSCT) system. Eur Radiol 2006;16(2):256–68.

3. Megibow AJ, Sahani D. Best practice: implementation and use of abdominal dual-energy CT in routine patient care. AJR Am J Roentgenol 2012;199(5 Suppl):S71–7.

4. Johnson TR, Krauss B, Sedlmair M, et al. Material differentiation by dual energy CT: initial experience. Eur Radiol 2007;17(6):1510–7.

5. Toepker M, Moritz T, Krauss B, et al. Virtual non-contrast in second-generation, dual-energy computed tomography: reliability of attenuation values. Eur J Radiol 2012;81(3):e398–405.

6. Slebocki K, Kraus B, Chang DH, et al. Incidental findings in abdominal dual-energy computed tomography: correlation between true noncontrast and virtual noncontrast images considering renal and liver cysts and adrenal masses. J Comput Assist Tomogr 2017;41(2):294–7.

7. Helck A, Hummel N, Meinel FG, et al. Can single-phase dual-energy CT reliably identify adrenal adenomas? Eur Radiol 2014;24(7):1636–42.

8. Chandarana H, Godoy MC, Vlahos I, et al. Abdominal aorta: evaluation with dual-source dual-energy multidetector CT after endovascular repair of aneurysms–initial observations. Radiology 2008; 249(2):692–700.

9. Sun H, Hou XY, Xue HD, et al. Dual-source dual-energy CT angiography with virtual non-enhanced images and iodine map for active gastrointestinal bleeding: image quality, radiation dose and diagnostic performance. Eur J Radiol 2015;84(5): 884–91.

10. Agrawal MD, Pinho DF, Kulkarni NM, et al. Oncologic applications of dual-energy CT in the abdomen. Radiographics 2014;34(3):589–612.

11. Lee JA, Jeong WK, Kim Y, et al. Dual-energy CT to detect recurrent HCC after TACE: initial experience of color-coded iodine CT imaging. Eur J Radiol 2013;82(4):569–76.

12. Chandarana H, Megibow AJ, Cohen BA, et al. Iodine quantification with dual-energy CT: phantom study and preliminary experience with renal masses. AJR Am J Roentgenol 2011;196(6):W693–700.

13. Pelgrim GJ, van Hamersvelt RW, Willemink MJ, et al. Accuracy of iodine quantification using dual energy CT in latest generation dual source and dual layer CT. Eur Radiol 2017;27(9):3904–12.

14. Chen X, Xu Y, Duan J, et al. Correlation of iodine uptake and perfusion parameters between dual-energy CT imaging and first-pass dual-input perfusion CT in lung cancer. Medicine (Baltimore) 2017; 96(28):e7479.

15. Stiller W, Skornitzke S, Fritz F, et al. Correlation of quantitative dual-energy computed tomography iodine maps and abdominal computed tomography perfusion measurements: are single-acquisition dual-energy computed tomography iodine maps more than a reduced-dose surrogate of conventional computed tomography perfusion? Invest Radiol 2015;50(10):703–8.

16. Grant KL, Flohr TG, Krauss B, et al. Assessment of an advanced image-based technique to calculate virtual monoenergetic computed tomographic images from a dual-energy examination to improve contrast-to-noise ratio in examinations using iodinated contrast media. Invest Radiol 2014;49(9): 586–92.

17. Michalak G, Grimes J, Fletcher J, et al. Technical note: improved CT number stability across patient size using dual-energy CT virtual monoenergetic imaging. Med Phys 2016;43(1):513.

18. Yu L, Leng S, McCollough CH. Dual-energy CT-based monochromatic imaging. AJR Am J Roentgenol 2012;199(5 Suppl):S9–15.

19. Mileto A, Barina A, Marin D, et al. Virtual monochromatic images from dual-energy multidetector CT: variance in CT numbers from the same lesion between single-source projection-based and dual-source image-based implementations. Radiology 2016;279(1):269–77.

20. Wichmann JL, Hardie AD, Schoepf UJ, et al. Single- and dual-energy CT of the abdomen: comparison of radiation dose and image quality of 2nd and 3rd generation dual-source CT. Eur Radiol 2017;27(2):642–50.

21. Uhrig M, Simons D, Kachelriess M, et al. Advanced abdominal imaging with dual energy CT is feasible without increasing radiation dose. Cancer Imaging 2016;16(1):15.

22. Silva AC, Morse BG, Hara AK, et al. Dual-energy (spectral) CT: applications in abdominal imaging. Radiographics 2011;31(4):1031–46 [discussion: 1047–50].

23. Kaza RK, Platt JF, Cohan RH, et al. Dual-energy CT with single- and dual-source scanners: current applications in evaluating the genitourinary tract. Radiographics 2012;32(2):353–69.

24. Morgan DE. Dual-energy CT of the abdomen. Abdom Imaging 2014;39(1):108–34.

25. Heye T, Nelson RC, Ho LM, et al. Dual-energy CT applications in the abdomen. AJR Am J Roentgenol 2012;199(5 Suppl):S64–70.

26. Patel BN, Alexander L, Allen B, et al. Dual-energy CT workflow: multi-institutional consensus on standardization of abdominopelvic MDCT protocols. Abdom Radiol (NY) 2017;42(3):676–87.

27. Bolus D, Morgan D, Berland L. Effective use of the Hounsfield unit in the age of variable energy CT. Abdom Radiol (NY) 2017;42(3):766–71.

28. Borhani AA, Kulzer M, Iranpour N, et al. Comparison of true unenhanced and virtual unenhanced (VUE) attenuation values in abdominopelvic single-source rapid kilovoltage-switching spectral CT. Abdom Radiol (NY) 2017;42(3):710–7.

29. Kaza RK, Caoili EM, Cohan RH, et al. Distinguishing enhancing from nonenhancing renal lesions with fast kilovoltage-switching dual-energy CT. AJR Am J Roentgenol 2011;197(6):1375–81.

30. Kaza RK, Ananthakrishnan L, Kambadakone A, et al. Update of dual-energy CT applications in the genitourinary tract. AJR Am J Roentgenol 2017;208(6):1185–92.

31. Zarzour JG, Milner D, Valentin R, et al. Quantitative iodine content threshold for discrimination of renal cell carcinomas using rapid kV-switching dual-energy CT. Abdom Radiol (NY) 2017;42(3):727–34.

32. Bongers MN, Schabel C, Krauss B, et al. Noise-optimized virtual monoenergetic images and iodine maps for the detection of venous thrombosis in second-generation dual-energy CT (DECT): an ex vivo phantom study. Eur Radiol 2015;25(6):1655–64.

33. Vandenbroucke F, Van Hedent S, Van Gompel G, et al. Dual-energy CT after radiofrequency ablation of liver, kidney, and lung lesions: a review of features. Insights Imaging 2015;6(3):363–79.

34. Kambadakone AR, Eisner BH, Catalano OA, et al. New and evolving concepts in the imaging and management of urolithiasis: urologists' perspective. Radiographics 2010;30(3):603–23.

35. Masch WR, Cronin KC, Sahani DV, et al. Imaging in urolithiasis. Radiol Clin North Am 2017;55(2):209–24.

36. Clark ZE, Bolus DN, Little MD, et al. Abdominal rapid-kVp-switching dual-energy MDCT with reduced IV contrast compared to conventional MDCT with standard weight-based IV contrast: an intra-patient comparison. Abdom Imaging 2015;40(4):852–8.

37. Euler A, Parakh A, Falkowski AL, et al. Initial results of a single-source dual-energy computed tomography technique using a split-filter: assessment of image quality, radiation dose, and accuracy of dual-energy applications in an in vitro and in vivo study. Invest Radiol 2016;51(8):491–8.

38. Ananthakrishnan L, Rajiah P, Ahn R, et al. Spectral detector CT-derived virtual non-contrast images: comparison of attenuation values with unenhanced CT. Abdom Radiol (NY) 2017;42(3):702–9.

39. McCollough CH, Leng S, Yu L, et al. Dual- and multi-energy CT: principles, technical approaches, and clinical applications. Radiology 2015;276(3):637–53.

40. Kaufmann S, Sauter A, Spira D, et al. Tin-filter enhanced dual-energy-CT: image quality and accuracy of CT numbers in virtual noncontrast imaging. Acad Radiol 2013;20(5):596–603.

41. Rassouli N, Chalian H, Rajiah P, et al. Assessment of 70-keV virtual monoenergetic spectral images in abdominal CT imaging: a comparison study to conventional polychromatic 120-kVp images. Abdom Radiol (NY) 2017;42(10):2579–86.

42. Wellenberg RH, Boomsma MF, van Osch JA, et al. Quantifying metal artefact reduction using virtual monochromatic dual-layer detector spectral CT imaging in unilateral and bilateral total hip prostheses. Eur J Radiol 2017;88:61–70.

43. Rajiah P, Abbara S, Halliburton SS. Spectral detector CT for cardiovascular applications. Diagn Interv Radiol 2017;23(3):187–93.

Dual-Energy Computed Tomography in Cardiothoracic Vascular Imaging

Domenico De Santis, MD[a,b], Marwen Eid, MD[a],
Carlo N. De Cecco, MD, PhD[a], Brian E. Jacobs, BS[a],
Moritz H. Albrecht, MD[a,c], Akos Varga-Szemes, MD, PhD[a],
Christian Tesche, MD[a,d], Damiano Caruso, MD[b],
Andrea Laghi, MD[b], Uwe Joseph Schoepf, MD[a,*]

KEYWORDS

- Dual energy computed tomography • Virtual monoenergetic images • Virtual noncontrast images
- Cardiac CT perfusion • Pulmonary CT perfusion • Calcium subtraction • Metal artifact reduction
- Plaque analysis

KEY POINTS

- The fundamental principle of dual energy computed tomography is the acquisition of 2 imaged datasets at low and high energy, enabling enhanced spectral information.
- The implementation of low keV virtual monoenergetic images allows for improved contrast characteristics, and high keV levels reduce blooming artifacts.
- Virtual noncontrast reconstructions can effectively replace true noncontrast acquisitions, reducing both radiation dose and scan time.
- Dual energy–based material decomposition can be used to selectively subtract materials from the image, which improves the overall diagnostic performance of computed tomography angiography examinations.
- Dual energy computed tomography can identify myocardial and pulmonary perfusion defects and holds the potential to noninvasively assess plaque composition, providing incremental information for patient management.

INTRODUCTION

Dual energy computed tomography (DECT) refers to the acquisition of CT data with 2 CT datasets at differing x-ray energy spectra.[1] Because different materials show differences in photon absorption at various energy levels, DECT allows for material decomposition and more accurate tissue characterization compared with single energy CT, the latter of which can only provide simple density-

Disclosures: Dr U.J. Schoepf is a consultant for and/or receives research support from Astellas, Bayer, GE, Guerbet, Medrad, and Siemens. Dr C.N. De Cecco receives research support from Siemens.

[a] Department of Radiology and Radiological Science, Division of Cardiovascular Imaging, Medical University of South Carolina, 25 Courtenay Drive, Charleston, SC 29425, USA; [b] Department of Radiological Sciences, Oncology and Pathology, University of Rome "Sapienza", Piazzale Aldo Moro 5, Rome 00185, Italy; [c] Department of Diagnostic and Interventional Radiology, University Hospital Frankfurt, Theodor-Stern-Kai 7, Frankfurt am Main 60590, Germany; [d] Department of Cardiology and Intensive Care Medicine, Heart Center Munich-Bogenhausen, Lazarettstraße 36, Munich 80636, Germany

* Corresponding author. Department of Radiology and Radiological Science, Medical University of South Carolina, 25 Courtenay Drive, Charleston, SC.

E-mail address: schoepf@musc.edu

Radiol Clin N Am 56 (2018) 521–534
https://doi.org/10.1016/j.rcl.2018.03.010

based morphologic assessment.[2] With the most recent advancements in CT technology, particularly increased spatial and temporal resolutions as well as improved tube voltage and radiation dose optimization strategies, near simultaneous acquisitions at 2 different energy spectra can be performed while maintaining or decreasing the radiation dose. As a result of these advancements, there was a renewed interest in the possible applications of DECT for cardiovascular imaging,[3] including the improvement of contrast conditions, virtual noncontrast images, metal artifact reduction, virtual calcium subtraction, parenchymal perfusion evaluation, and improved tissue characterization.

The aim of this article is to provide an overview of well-established DECT investigational and technical solutions applied to cardiothoracic vascular imaging.

Dual Energy Computed Tomography: Technical Approaches

DECT scanner manufacturers have developed different technical strategies to obtain dual energy image datasets. Currently, there are 6 types of DECT scanners:

1. Single-source helical DECT (Siemens Healthineers, Forchheim, Germany);
2. Single-source sequential DECT (Toshiba, Tochigi, Japan);
3. Single-source fast kVp switching DECT (GE Healthcare, Milwaukee, WI);
4. Single-source twin-beam DECT (Siemens Healthineers);
5. Dual source DECT (Siemens Healthineers); and
6. Dual-layer DECT (Philips Healthcare, Best, the Netherlands)

Regardless of each scanner's technical approach to data acquisition, the fundamental principle of DECT and overall goal of the various technical solutions remains the same: to simultaneously obtain and analyze data characterized by 2 different x-ray energy levels.

Dual Energy Computed Tomography: Image Postprocessing

Material decomposition
The attenuation values measured in dual energy at the 2 varying energy spectra allow the assessment of the chemical composition of tissues. Different algorithms have been implemented to achieve material decomposition, either in the prereconstruction (projection) space or in the image domain.[1,4] As result, it is possible to generate additional image sets by generating a color-coded iodine map

or selectively subtracting a specific material from the data, similar to what is displayed in virtual non-contrast and virtual calcium-subtracted images.

Blended images
The DECT-derived dataset routinely used for clinical purposes consists of high and low kVp data blended together to obtain CT images similar to the conventional polyenergetic single energy CT images.[5] Although different blending techniques have been developed to obtain the final images, the most common approach consists of a linear blend between high and low kVp datasets using different blend percentages. However, data can also be blended with a nonlinear technique, the so-called sigmoidal blending, which ultimately leads to an improved contrast resolution.[6] Focusing on cardiovascular applications, sigmoidal blended images outperformed traditional linearly blended datasets in the detection of acute myocardial infarct[7] and in the identification of left ventricular late iodine enhancement, a conventional landmark of chronic myocardial infarct.[8]

Virtual monoenergetic images
Despite the well-established role of blended images, one of the most promising applications of DECT is the potential to generate virtual monoenergetic images (VMI).[9] VMI can be generated in either the projection domain (implemented by single source fast kVp switching scanners) or the image domain (implemented by dual source dual energy scanners).[10] Notably, VMI have the potential to reduce beam hardening artifacts more than traditional techniques used on linearly blended images. In terms of image quality, VMI have been evaluated extensively in recent years, with results suggesting that optimal image quality is obtained with acquisitions performed at 70 keV.[11,12] In 2014, Grant and colleagues[13] introduced a new image-based method that enables the calculation of VMI images from dual source dual energy examinations. This technique, termed VMI+, combines data from low keV images with data from higher keV levels. Inherently, low keV scans are characterized by increased contrast and image noise, whereas high keV acquisitions are characterized by optimal image noise but inferior contrast. Thus, the data are decomposed in an advantageous manner to capitalize on the unique capabilities afforded by acquisitions at different keV levels. Specifically, the high contrast ratio is used from the low keV data and the optimal image noise is used from the high keV data.

As a result, the algorithm generates VMI+, which is characterized by significantly lower image noise compared with VMI at every monoenergetic level. Therefore, this technique is attractive for clinical use, because low keV VMI+ images (40–50 keV) provide the highest image quality. To date, dual source DECT data can be processed to generate a spectrum of VMI+ images, ranging from 40 to 190 keV at 1 keV increments. This allows the radiologist to select the most suitable dataset from a broad spectrum of images for the diagnostic purpose at hand.

CLINICAL APPLICATIONS
Improved Image Contrast

Perhaps the most common problem faced during CT angiography examination is poor contrast within the vessels. Traditionally, iodine attenuation values ranging from 250 to 350 Hounsfield units are considered adequate to achieve diagnostic image quality within the vessel.[14] To counteract the risk of inadequate vessel opacification, the only viable option with single energy CT scanners is to reduce the tube voltage to emphasize the iodine attenuation. However, such an approach is limited by the concomitant increase of image noise, which can noticeably hamper diagnostic accuracy, especially in vascular districts characterized by complex anatomy and tiny vessels. However, the implementation of VMI at low keV in DECT improves the depiction of all vessels, especially in the small peripheral branches.[15]

In fact, such datasets are particularly effective in vascular studies, in which the importance of high contrast typically outweighs the desire for low image noise.[16] Recently, a comprehensive analysis[17] of VMI applied to thoracoabdominal DECT angiography demonstrated that VMI+ series at 40 to 50 keV provide the greatest objective image quality and offer improved visualization of tiny arterial branches compared with the traditional monoenergetic algorithm. These results have been further strengthened by additional investigations demonstrating that 40 keV VMI+ substantially improves the evaluation of patients scheduled for transcatheter aortic valve replacement.[18] In addition, studies have demonstrated that VMI+ reconstructions hold the potential to play a role in postinterventional coronary evaluation. Compared with traditional algorithms, results suggest that VMI+ reconstructions offer improved lumen visualization in stents that are 3 mm or smaller, with optimal results obtained at 130 keV.[19] Furthermore, VMI reconstructions at low keV levels are beneficial for identifying chronic myocardial infarction from delayed enhancement DECT[20] (Fig. 1) and increasing the accuracy of stress DECT perfusion in detecting perfusion defects.[21] Notably, perfusion defects showed

significantly greater attenuation differences at lower keV levels, with the greatest difference seen at 40 keV, reaching a sensitivity and specificity of 96% and 98%, respectively.

With regard to the pulmonary vessels, CT pulmonary angiography is paramount in cases of suspected pulmonary embolism (PE).[22] In fact, an accurate diagnosis of PE is crucial, because it directly impacts downstream patient management. To achieve an accurate diagnosis, particularly with smaller subsegmental emboli, contrast conditions must be optimal. However, often times CT pulmonary angiography results in suboptimal contrast enhancement. This is typically caused by poor bolus tracking timing, breathing-related motion artifacts, and low cardiac output, rendering the diagnosis of PE inconclusive.[23] Therefore, monoenergetic reconstructions have the potential to provide additional diagnostic value in the detection and classification of PE. By reconstructing images at low keV levels (<60 keV), contrast conditions of an initially suboptimal examination can be greatly improved, effectively enhancing the ability to visualize smaller vessels and detect emboli in the pulmonary vasculature[17,24] (Fig. 2). A recent study[25] evaluated the use of VMI+ and iodine perfusion maps from chest DECT for the detection of PE in examinations with suboptimal contrast enhancement, concluding that the additional assessment of virtual monoenergetic reconstructions provided improved diagnostic accuracy in PE detection. In addition, it has been demonstrated that the use of 40 keV VMI+ can help to diagnose incidental PE in oncologic patients undergoing portal–venous phase DECT, effectively turning a venous acquisition into an arterial scan.[26] Other than enhancing the ability to detect PE, low keV monoenergetic image reconstructions improve contrast conditions in the thoracic aorta, which are typically suboptimal in pulmonary angiography studies. The improved contrast in the aorta increases the ability of radiologists to detect incidental findings, such as aortic dissection.[27] Moreover, the use of DECT at low keV with iodine maps allows for improved visualization and tracking of potential endoleaks after stent treatment for aortic dissection or aneurysm.[28] Last, but certainly not least, low keV VMI has the theoretic capacity to reduce the contrast media volume needed to reach vascular diagnostic attenuation values.[15,29]

Virtual Noncontrast Images

Coronary CT angiography (CCTA) is a reliable, noninvasive imaging modality for coronary artery assessment in patients with an intermediate

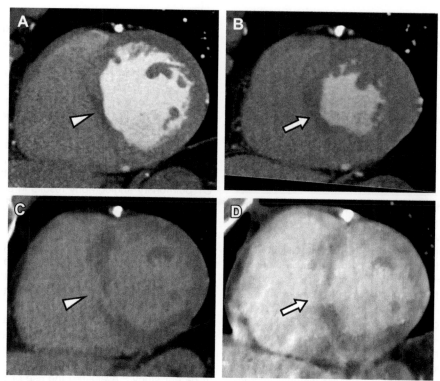

Fig. 1. Dual energy myocardial computed tomography perfusion in a 67-year-old man presenting with chest pain. Rest (*A, arrowhead*) and stress phase (*B, arrow*) show a fixed myocardial perfusion defect of the septal left ventricular wall. Delayed enhancement was obtained by mixed linearly blended reconstruction (*C, arrowhead*) and shows septal hyperenhancement that is better delineated with VMI+ reconstructions at 40 keV (*D, arrow*).

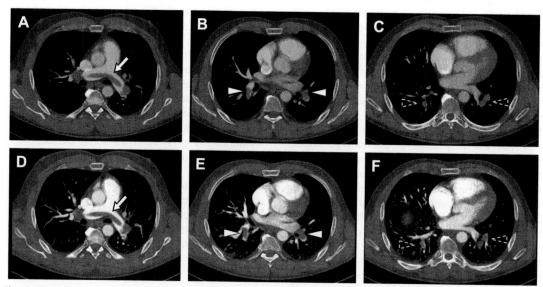

Fig. 2. Dual energy pulmonary computed tomography perfusion in a 55-year-old woman with chest pain and shortness of breath. Linearly blended reconstructions show a pulmonary saddle embolus (*A, arrow*) as well as bilateral subsegmental emboli (*B, arrowheads; C, dashed arrowheads*). VMI+ reconstructions at 40 keV improve contrast within the pulmonary arteries, better depicting the saddle embolus (*D, arrow*) and the bilateral subsegmental emboli (*E, arrowhead; F, dashed arrowheads*).

pretest probability of coronary artery disease.[30] In such a clinical scenario, a fundamental procedure in the diagnosis of coronary disease is the calcium score (CaSc). This procedure, characterized by the quantification of coronary calcium, is paramount to patient risk stratification. CaSc data are typically obtained with a noncontrast CT acquisition performed before the angiographic phase of the scan. Despite the undoubted clinical usefulness, this technique results in a slight increase to both acquisition time and radiation dose.[31] Interestingly, radiation dose concerns were partly responsible for the downgraded status of the CaSc in the American College of Cardiology/American Heart Association Guideline on the Assessment of Cardiovascular Risk. Specifically, in 2013, the CaSc was demoted from a class IIA recommendation to class IIB in asymptomatic patients with intermediate risk.[32]

Through virtual noncontrast images, DECT is able to generate a dataset characterized by a virtual iodine removal, which is theoretically suitable for CaSc calculation (**Fig. 3**). Schwarz and colleagues[33] pioneered investigations focusing on the potential for virtual noncontrast images generated by a dual source DECT system to be used in the calculation of CaSc and calcium volume, demonstrating that calcium volume in the virtual noncontrast dataset, although slightly underestimated, had excellent correlation with values obtained from the true noncontrast images. Results from this study were later strengthened by other investigations[34,35] that confirmed the excellent correlation between virtual noncontrast and true noncontrast datasets. Eventually, the DECT angiography protocol demonstrated to be dose effective compared with the single energy examination (4.3 ± 0.3 vs 5.4 ± 0.7 mSv).[34]

However, all of these studies[33–35] elucidated the slight underestimation of calcium values provided by the virtual noncontrast dataset compared with the traditional single energy dataset, which was specifically adopted for CaSc purposes. It is plausible that these discrepant values may be the result of less beam hardening and blooming artifacts encountered in the dual energy datasets. Thus, the possibility that virtual noncontrast values may represent more accurate calcium quantification should be taken into account. Further investigations correlating virtual noncontrast findings with ex vivo calcified coronary plaques are required.

Another interesting application of virtual noncontrast images in cardiothoracic vascular imaging is the evaluation of endoleaks after aortic endovascular repair. The traditional acquisition protocol consists of a true noncontrast acquisition followed by arterial and delayed phases. Virtual noncontrast images generated with DECT datasets can effectively replace the true noncontrast acquisition, providing high diagnostic accuracy for the detection of endoleaks and significant radiation dose reductions of more than 60%.[36]

Calcium Subtraction Images

Bony structures and extensive vascular calcifications are responsible for blooming artifacts and consequently hinder the accurate evaluation of vascular territories. Moreover, these structures, characterized by high atomic densities, are always represented in multiplanar reformatting images, which are routinely used in clinical practice for the evaluation of CT angiography owing to their ability to provide an immediate overview of the vascular territory.

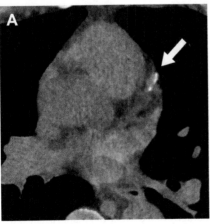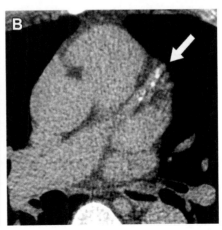

Fig. 3. Dual energy coronary computed tomography angiography in a 59-year-old man with acute chest pain. Virtual noncontrast image reveals calcified plaques in the left anterior descending coronary artery (*A, arrow*). The corresponding true unenhanced calcium scoring scan confirms the calcified coronary plaque (*B, arrow*).

Postprocessing techniques for calcium subtraction in single energy CT are based on threshold-growing algorithms, which are time consuming and require manual corrections. Other single energy CT techniques dedicated to bone removal are based on a double acquisition. Specifically, acquisitions are performed before and after contrast media administration to generate calcium-subtracted images in a similar manner to digital subtraction angiography. However, this solution is significantly hampered by misregistration artifacts, which reduce the overall image quality and prevent accurate diagnosis. Further, the double exposure fundamental to this approach leads to an increased radiation dose.[37,38]

In contrast, DECT has the ability to quantify and delineate calcium from iodine based on their differing mass attenuation coefficients when interacting with high and low kVp spectra. As a result, virtual calcium-subtracted images generated from DECT datasets can be obtained within a single CT phase by means of dedicated algorithms. This effectively removes the need for multiple acquisitions and curtails the risk of image misalignments and increased radiation dose (Fig. 4). Several investigations have suggested that DECT-based calcium-subtracted images outperform single energy derived images, providing an improved depiction of vessel lumen in several vascular territories.[39–41] Nevertheless, dual energy–based calcium subtraction techniques are hampered by lower efficacies in vascular territories with tiny vessels.[41,42] To overcome this limitation, a modified material decomposition algorithm specifically developed to obtain calcium-subtracted images is currently a topic of active investigation. So far, this algorithm has demonstrated its feasibility with good preliminary results in the assessment of the supraaortic vessel[43] and coronary arteries.[44]

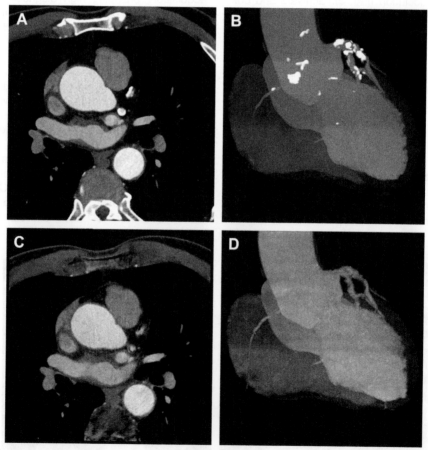

Fig. 4. Dual energy coronary computed tomography angiography in a 81-year-old man. Axial (A) and maximum intensity projection (B) images show heavily calcified coronary arteries. Corresponding images processed with dual energy calcium subtraction algorithm achieved complete calcium removal yielding better visualization of the coronary tree (C, D).

Metallic Artifact Reduction

The image quality of single energy CT datasets is hampered by metallic devices, which can cause severe beam hardening and photon starvation artifacts. However, both of these artifacts have a physical explanation and are intrinsically related to the polychromatic nature of the single energy x-ray beam. In particular, beam hardening is the result of a certain structure absorbing a higher percentage of low-energy photons compared with high-energy photons. This phenomenon causes the x-ray beam to appear harder than the others and is often characterized by dark bands or streaks across the image. Photon starvation artifacts, however, are related to the low amount of photons reaching the detectors, which ultimately leads to increased image noise.[45] Previous strategies used to reduce beam hardening artifacts relied on the development of specific algorithms and the use of higher tube potentials.[46] However, both strategies have specific disadvantages. Specifically, the former can lead to the development of new artifacts, and the latter causes an increase in radiation dose.[47]

DECT-derived VMI at high keV levels can reduce beam hardening artifacts with a mere postprocessing procedure by simply adjusting the monoenergetic level to the optimal value (Fig. 5). Bamberg and colleagues[46] were able to demonstrate in 31 patients with metallic implants who had undergone DECT that monoenergetic levels ranging from 95 to 150 keV provided superior image quality and diagnostic value compared with lower energy levels. Moreover, the implementation of such high energy levels made it possible to discern decisive diagnostic features that would have otherwise been missed. Meinel and colleagues[48] further strengthened these results by defining a dedicated dual source CT protocol and endorsing photon energies of 105 to 120 keV as the optimal range for metal artifact reduction.

Myocardial Perfusion

CCTA has been validated as a reliable tool for the detection of coronary artery disease in patients presenting with chest pain. However, determining the hemodynamic significance of a stenotic lesion identified on CCTA remains a challenge, because traditional CCTA provides anatomic rather than functional information.[49] Despite this initial limitation, DECT can be a valuable tool for the functional assessment of coronary artery disease, because it permits the generation of color-coded iodine perfusion maps for the visualization and quantification of myocardial iodine uptake, an indirect marker of myocardial perfusion.[3] Since its initial description in 2008,[50] this technique remains one of the most extensively investigated applications of cardiac DECT and has spurred an increased interest within the academic community.[51–54] DECT perfusion is typically performed at both rest and under pharmacologically induced stress conditions and results from a single snapshot of the myocardium at a single time point (Fig. 6). Areas of hypoattenuation indicate a perfusion defect; however, the classification of this defect depends on the phase in which it is visualized. For instance, hypoattenuating myocardium present only in the stress phase suggests reversible ischemia, whereas a perfusion defect at rest is suggestive of myocardial infarction. A delayed phase dataset can be acquired 8 to 10 minutes after perfusion to evaluate late myocardial enhancement (expression of myocardial fibrosis); however, its added diagnostic value remains questionable, because it corresponds with an increased radiation dose.[55] A recent investigation assessed the added

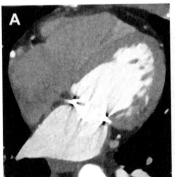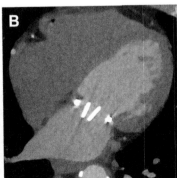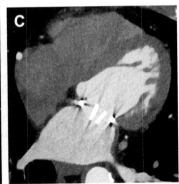

Fig. 5. Dual energy coronary computed tomography angiography in a 66-year-old woman after mitral valve replacement surgery. VMI+ reconstructions at 40 keV (A), 100 keV (B), and linearly blended images (C) show different degrees of blooming artifacts of the artificial mitral valve. The 100 keV VMI+ dataset yields lower artifacts than lower energy levels and blended images.

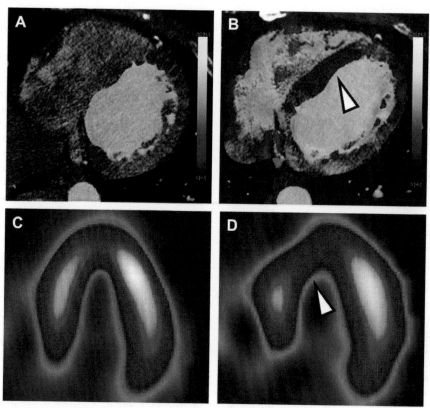

Fig. 6. Dual energy myocardial computed tomography (DECT) perfusion scan of a 62-year-old man. Rest phase (*A*) seems to be normal, whereas the iodine map at stress phase (*B*) unveils a reversible perfusion defect in the anteroseptal wall (*arrowhead*). Single photon emission computed tomography images at rest and stress (*C, D*) confirm the DECT finding (*D, arrowhead*).

value of stress DECT myocardial perfusion on standard CCTA, demonstrating that the combination of the 2 methods outperforms mere morphologic CCTA evaluation in the identification of significant coronary artery stenosis.[53] In addition to the purely visual assessment of myocardial perfusion, DECT iodine maps allow for the quantification of myocardial iodine uptake by providing values in milligrams per milliliter (**Fig. 7**).[1] A recent investigation aimed to quantify myocardial iodine uptake at stress DECT perfusion to discriminate between healthy and pathologic myocardium. Results suggested that an optimal threshold concentration of 2.1 mg of iodine per milliliter serves to delineate between healthy and diseased myocardium. Nevertheless, myocardial ischemia, situated between the thresholds for necrosis and normality, returned an overlap in iodine uptake values and, thus, requires further investigation to strengthen and refine these results.[56] Notably, it is important to exercise caution when interpreting these values, because a lack of standardization among the different DECT vendors raises reproducibility concerns.

Pulmonary Perfusion

Through material decomposition and the generation of pulmonary iodine distribution maps, it is possible to quantify the perfused blood volume (PBV) and investigate the presence of perfusion defects, further enhancing the diagnostic accuracy of DECT in the detection of PE and other abnormalities.[24,25,57–59] Perfusion maps provide functional and prognostic information in addition to the purely anatomic assessment of pulmonary vessel lumen. Reduced lung perfusion can be visualized as decreased iodine uptake in the affected area, whereas pulmonary infarct is represented by a peripheral wedge-shaped perfusion defect correlating with lung scintigraphy.[60] The addition of PBV maps to CT pulmonary angiography increases the diagnostic accuracy of intrapulmonary clots in patients with suspected PE (**Fig. 8**).[61] PBV quantification also has an impact on patient management and prognosis.[62,63] In particular, Meinel and colleagues[64] demonstrated a significant negative correlation between global PBV values, the Qanadli score, and the right-to-

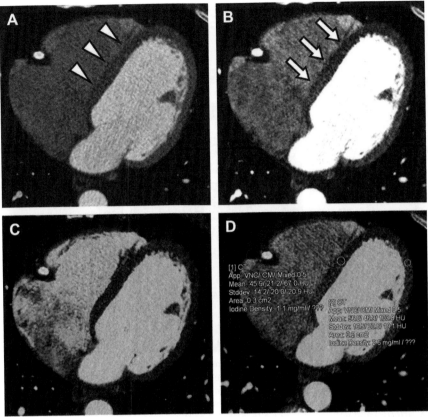

Fig. 7. Dual energy myocardial computed tomography perfusion scan of a 58-year-old woman. Stress acquisition reconstructed by means of linearly blended images reveals a perfusion defect of the septal wall (*A, arrowheads*), which is better visualized by 40 keV VMI+ reconstructions (*B, arrows*). Iodine maps at rest (*C*) and stress phases (*D*) allows for precise iodine quantification, confirming the presence of a reversible myocardial perfusion defect.

left ventricle diameter ratio. Additionally, patients with a PBV value of less than 60% were associated with a significantly higher risk of requiring intensive care unit admission compared with individuals with a PBV of 60% or greater.[64] Another interesting application of DECT in the setting of pulmonary disease is xenon-enhanced DECT ventilation. This technique was shown to be feasible; however, it remains in early experimental stages.[65]

Pulmonary Hypertension

DECT can play an important role in the noninvasive diagnosis of chronic thromboembolic pulmonary hypertension.[66] By providing perfusion and angiographic information within a single examination, this imaging technique has a sensitivity and specificity of 100% and 92% in the diagnosis of chronic thromboembolic pulmonary hypertension, respectively. In particular, DECT perfusion outperforms CT angiography in the identification of segmental abnormalities.[67] Moreover, DECT can be used to quantify pulmonary artery and whole lung enhancement values (higher and lower in

chronic thromboembolic pulmonary hypertension patients compared with healthy individuals, respectively). The derived central-to-peripheral ratio (10.9 vs 8.4 in patients with chronic thromboembolic pulmonary hypertension and healthy subjects, respectively) can help the radiologist to identify chronic thromboembolic pulmonary hypertension.[68]

Improved Tissue Characterization

It is well-known that the risk of plaque rupture is associated with its composition. Specifically, soft plaques containing lipid and necrotic parts are more likely to rupture than hard fibrotic plaques. Single energy CT only relies on Hounsfield unit measurement, and if there is any attenuation overlap among the different plaque components, such an assessment would not accurately reflect plaque composition.[2] In contrast, DECT tissue characterization is based on different material attenuation properties at high and low energy spectra. Therefore, this technique can theoretically serve as a method to achieve in vivo noninvasive plaque

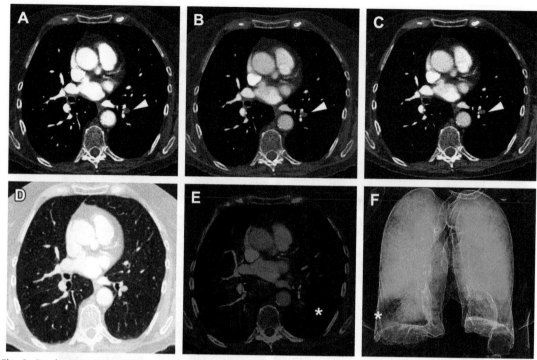

Fig. 8. Dual energy computed tomography (DECT) pulmonary angiography in a 72-year-old woman presenting with shortness of breath. VMI+ reconstructions at 40 keV (*A, arrowhead*) and 55 keV (*B, arrowhead*) reveal an embolus of a segmental pulmonary artery and provide improved contrast compared with linearly blended images (*C, arrowhead*). Axial view with lung windowing (*D*) reveals no wedge-shaped peripheral hyperdensity of the lungs. Axial (*E, asterisk*) and volume rendering (*F, asterisk*) of DECT lung perfusion unveils a defect of the posterior right lower lobe.

composition analysis. Good results have been reported by Obaid and colleagues,[69] who were able to distinguish the necrotic core from the fibrous cap with DECT examination, improving the proper management of vulnerable plaques. However, other investigations only found significant image patterns between calcified and noncalcified plaques, without statistical differences among the different subtypes of noncalcified plaques, such as fibrotic, lipid rich, and necrotic.[70] Further investigations and large prospective trials are needed to extensively assess DECT plaque analysis and obtain robust results.

New Frontiers of Dual Energy Computed Tomography in Cardiovascular Imaging

Although these applications have been the most extensively studied, DECT allows for additional applications that are still in early experimental phases.

It is a known fact that coronary plaque characteristics play in important role in the risk of experiencing a major adverse cardiac event. Single energy CT has demonstrated feasibility for plaque characteristic analysis, finding an association between plaque composition and the risk of major

adverse cardiac event[71,72] and in-stent restenosis.[73] However, through its material decomposition properties, DECT would allow for more accurate plaque characterization, thus providing additional information on plaque vulnerability and potentially improving major adverse cardiac event prediction and risk stratification.[69,74,75]

Another potential application of DECT is the calculation of extracellular volume fraction. The extracellular volume fraction is an indicator of myocardial fibrosis and, although this factor has previously been elucidated with MR imaging data, new evidence suggests that the extracellular volume fraction can be derived from DECT acquisitions.[76,77]

Finally, myocardial iron quantification with DECT has been shown to be feasible in patients with thalassemia, compared with MR imaging-based quantification as the reference standard. This may prove to be an important finding, because iron overload is the most important cause of death in this population of patients.[78]

SUMMARY

DECT allows for several applications in cardiothoracic vascular imaging that have been continuously translating from research to clinical practice. Therefore, DECT represents a cutting-edge technology that enables the use of various assessments that go far beyond the traditional concepts of material density. Cardiothoracic vascular imaging, owing to its intrinsically challenging nature, represents one of the most innovative fields of DECT technical development. This field of imaging has been radically changed by the implementation of such technology and further advancements are expected in the future.

REFERENCES

1. Siegel MJ, Kaza RK, Bolus DN, et al. White paper of the society of computed body tomography and magnetic resonance on dual-energy CT, part 1: technology and terminology. J Comput Assist Tomogr 2016;40(6):841–5.
2. Sun J, Zhang Z, Lu B, et al. Identification and quantification of coronary atherosclerotic plaques: a comparison of 64-MDCT and intravascular ultrasound. AJR Am J Roentgenol 2008;190(3):748–54.
3. Vliegenthart R, Pelgrim GJ, Ebersberger U, et al. Dual-energy CT of the heart. AJR Am J Roentgenol 2012;199(5 Suppl):S54–63.
4. McCollough CH, Leng S, Yu L, et al. Dual- and multi-energy CT: principles, technical approaches, and clinical applications. Radiology 2015;276(3):637–53.
5. Behrendt FF, Schmidt B, Plumhans C, et al. Image fusion in dual energy computed tomography: effect on contrast enhancement, signal-to-noise ratio and image quality in computed tomography angiography. Invest Radiol 2009;44(1):1–6.
6. Holmes DR 3rd, Fletcher JG, Apel A, et al. Evaluation of non-linear blending in dual-energy computed tomography. Eur J Radiol 2008;68(3):409–13.
7. Kartje JK, Schmidt B, Bruners P, et al. Dual energy CT with nonlinear image blending improves visualization of delayed myocardial contrast enhancement in acute myocardial infarction. Invest Radiol 2013; 48(1):41–5.
8. Wichmann JL, Hu X, Kerl JM, et al. Non-linear blending of dual-energy CT data improves depiction of late iodine enhancement in chronic myocardial infarction. Int J Cardiovasc Imaging 2014;30(6): 1145–50.
9. Alvarez RE, Macovski A. Energy-selective reconstructions in X-ray computerized tomography. Phys Med Biol 1976;21(5):733–44.
10. Yu L, Leng S, McCollough CH. Dual-energy CT-based monochromatic imaging. AJR Am J Roentgenol 2012;199(5 Suppl):S9–15.
11. Apfaltrer P, Sudarski S, Schneider D, et al. Value of monoenergetic low-kV dual energy CT datasets for improved image quality of CT pulmonary angiography. Eur J Radiol 2014;83(2):322–8.
12. Schneider D, Apfaltrer P, Sudarski S, et al. Optimization of kiloelectron volt settings in cerebral and cervical dual-energy CT angiography determined with virtual monoenergetic imaging. Acad Radiol 2014; 21(4):431–6.
13. Grant KL, Flohr TG, Krauss B, et al. Assessment of an advanced image-based technique to calculate virtual monoenergetic computed tomographic images from a dual-energy examination to improve contrast-to-noise ratio in examinations using iodinated contrast media. Invest Radiol 2014;49(9): 586–92.
14. Becker CR, Hong C, Knez A, et al. Optimal contrast application for cardiac 4-detector-row computed tomography. Invest Radiol 2003;38(11):690–4.
15. Yuan R, Shuman WP, Earls JP, et al. Reduced iodine load at CT pulmonary angiography with dual-energy monochromatic imaging: comparison with standard CT pulmonary angiography–a prospective randomized trial. Radiology 2012;262(1):290–7.
16. Kalra MK, Rizzo S, Maher MM, et al. Chest CT performed with z-axis modulation: scanning protocol and radiation dose. Radiology 2005;237(1):303–8.
17. Albrecht MH, Trommer J, Wichmann JL, et al. Comprehensive comparison of virtual monoenergetic and linearly blended reconstruction techniques in third-generation dual-source dual-energy computed tomography angiography of the thorax and abdomen. Invest Radiol 2016;51(9):582–90.
18. Martin SS, Albrecht MH, Wichmann JL, et al. Value of a noise-optimized virtual monoenergetic reconstruction technique in dual-energy CT for planning of transcatheter aortic valve replacement. Eur Radiol 2017;27(2):705–14.
19. Mangold S, Cannao PM, Schoepf UJ, et al. Impact of an advanced image-based monoenergetic reconstruction algorithm on coronary stent visualization using third generation dual-source dual-energy CT: a phantom study. Eur Radiol 2016;26(6):1871–8.
20. Wichmann JL, Arbaciauskaite R, Kerl JM, et al. Evaluation of monoenergetic late iodine enhancement dual-energy computed tomography for imaging of chronic myocardial infarction. Eur Radiol 2014; 24(6):1211–8.
21. Carrascosa P, Deviggiano A, de Zan M, et al. Improved discrimination of myocardial perfusion defects at low energy levels using virtual monochromatic imaging. J Comput Assist Tomogr 2017; 41(4):661–7.
22. Stein PD, Fowler SE, Goodman LR, et al. Multidetector computed tomography for acute pulmonary embolism. N Engl J Med 2006;354(22):2317–27.
23. Jones SE, Wittram C. The indeterminate CT pulmonary angiogram: imaging characteristics and patient clinical outcome. Radiology 2005;237(1):329–37.
24. Albrecht MH, Bickford MW, Nance JW Jr, et al. State-of-the-art pulmonary CT angiography for acute

pulmonary embolism. AJR Am J Roentgenol 2017; 208(3):495–504.

25. Leithner D, Wichmann JL, Vogl TJ, et al. Virtual monoenergetic imaging and iodine perfusion maps improve diagnostic accuracy of dual-energy computed tomography pulmonary angiography with suboptimal contrast attenuation. Invest Radiol 2017;52(11):659–65.

26. Weiss J, Notohamiprodjo M, Bongers M, et al. Effect of noise-optimized monoenergetic postprocessing on diagnostic accuracy for detecting incidental pulmonary embolism in portal-venous phase dual-energy computed tomography. Invest Radiol 2017; 52(3):142–7.

27. Godoy MC, Naidich DP, Marchiori E, et al. Single-acquisition dual-energy multidetector computed tomography: analysis of vascular enhancement and postprocessing techniques for evaluating the thoracic aorta. J Comput Assist Tomogr 2010; 34(5):670–7.

28. Stolzmann P, Frauenfelder T, Pfammatter T, et al. Endoleaks after endovascular abdominal aortic aneurysm repair: detection with dual-energy dual-source CT. Radiology 2008;249(2):682–91.

29. Foley WD, Shuman WP, Siegel MJ, et al. White paper of the society of computed body tomography and magnetic resonance on dual-energy CT, part 2: radiation dose and iodine sensitivity. J Comput Assist Tomogr 2016;40(6):846–50.

30. Rubin GD, Leipsic J, Joseph Schoepf U, et al. CT angiography after 20 years: a transformation in cardiovascular disease characterization continues to advance. Radiology 2014;271(3):633–52.

31. Kim KP, Einstein AJ, Berrington de Gonzalez A. Coronary artery calcification screening: estimated radiation dose and cancer risk. Arch Intern Med 2009; 169(13):1188–94.

32. Goff DC Jr, Lloyd-Jones DM, Bennett G, et al. 2013 ACC/AHA guideline on the assessment of cardiovascular risk: a report of the American College of Cardiology/American Heart Association task force on practice guidelines. J Am Coll Cardiol 2014; 63(25 Pt B):2935–59.

33. Schwarz F, Nance JW Jr, Ruzsics B, et al. Quantification of coronary artery calcium on the basis of dual-energy coronary CT angiography. Radiology 2012; 264(3):700–7.

34. Yamada Y, Jinzaki M, Okamura T, et al. Feasibility of coronary artery calcium scoring on virtual unenhanced images derived from single-source fast kVp-switching dual-energy coronary CT angiography. J Cardiovasc Comput Tomogr 2014;8(5): 391–400.

35. Song I, Yi JG, Park JH, et al. Virtual non-contrast CT using dual-energy spectral CT: feasibility of coronary artery calcium scoring. Korean J Radiol 2016;17(3): 321–9.

36. De Cecco CN, Schoepf UJ, Steinbach L, et al. White paper of the society of computed body tomography and magnetic resonance on dual-energy CT, part 3: vascular, cardiac, pulmonary, and musculoskeletal applications. J Comput Assist Tomogr 2017;41(1):1–7.

37. Yoshioka K, Tanaka R, Muranaka K, et al. Subtraction coronary CT angiography using second-generation 320-detector row CT. Int J Cardiovasc Imaging 2015;31(suppl 1):51–8.

38. Yoshioka K, Tanaka R, Muranaka K. Subtraction coronary CT angiography for calcified lesions. Cardiol Clin 2012;30(1):93–102.

39. Morhard D, Fink C, Graser A, et al. Cervical and cranial computed tomographic angiography with automated bone removal: dual energy computed tomography versus standard computed tomography. Invest Radiol 2009;44(5):293–7.

40. Deng K, Liu C, Ma R, et al. Clinical evaluation of dual-energy bone removal in CT angiography of the head and neck: comparison with conventional bone-subtraction CT angiography. Clin Radiol 2009;64(5):534–41.

41. Meyer BC, Werncke T, Hopfenmuller W, et al. Dual energy CT of peripheral arteries: effect of automatic bone and plaque removal on image quality and grading of stenoses. Eur J Radiol 2008;68(3): 414–22.

42. Tran DN, Straka M, Roos JE, et al. Dual-energy CT discrimination of iodine and calcium: experimental results and implications for lower extremity CT angiography. Acad Radiol 2009;16(2):160–71.

43. Mannil M, Ramachandran J, Vittoria de Martini I, et al. Modified dual-energy algorithm for calcified plaque removal: evaluation in carotid computed tomography angiography and comparison with digital subtraction angiography. Invest Radiol 2017;52(11): 680–5.

44. De Santis D, Jin KN, Schoepf UJ, et al. Heavily calcified coronary arteries: advanced calcium subtraction improves luminal visualization and diagnostic confidence in dual-energy coronary computed tomography angiography. Invest Radiol 2018;53(2): 103–9.

45. Barrett JF, Keat N. Artifacts in CT: recognition and avoidance. Radiographics 2004;24(6):1679–91.

46. Bamberg F, Dierks A, Nikolaou K, et al. Metal artifact reduction by dual energy computed tomography using monoenergetic extrapolation. Eur Radiol 2011; 21(7):1424–9.

47. Watzke O, Kalender WA. A pragmatic approach to metal artifact reduction in CT: merging of metal artifact reduced images. Eur Radiol 2004;14(5):849–56.

48. Meinel FG, Bischoff B, Zhang Q, et al. Metal artifact reduction by dual-energy computed tomography using energetic extrapolation: a systematically optimized protocol. Invest Radiol 2012;47(7):406–14.

49. De Cecco CN, Varga-Szemes A, Meinel FG, et al. Beyond stenosis detection: computed tomography approaches for determining the functional relevance of coronary artery disease. Radiol Clin North Am 2015;53(2):317–34.

50. Ruzsics B, Lee H, Powers ER, et al. Images in cardiovascular medicine. Myocardial ischemia diagnosed by dual-energy computed tomography: correlation with single-photon emission computed tomography. Circulation 2008;117(9):1244–5.

51. Koonce JD, Vliegenthart R, Schoepf UJ, et al. Accuracy of dual-energy computed tomography for the measurement of iodine concentration using cardiac CT protocols: validation in a phantom model. Eur Radiol 2014;24(2):512–8.

52. Weininger M, Schoepf UJ, Ramachandra A, et al. Adenosine-stress dynamic real-time myocardial perfusion CT and adenosine-stress first-pass dual-energy myocardial perfusion CT for the assessment of acute chest pain: initial results. Eur J Radiol 2012; 81(12):3703–10.

53. De Cecco CN, Harris BS, Schoepf UJ, et al. Incremental value of pharmacological stress cardiac dual-energy CT over coronary CT angiography alone for the assessment of coronary artery disease in a high-risk population. AJR Am J Roentgenol 2014; 203(1):W70–7.

54. Ruzsics B, Lee H, Zwerner PL, et al. Dual-energy CT of the heart for diagnosing coronary artery stenosis and myocardial ischemia-initial experience. Eur Radiol 2008;18(11):2414–24.

55. Meinel FG, De Cecco CN, Schoepf UJ, et al. First-arterial-pass dual-energy CT for assessment of myocardial blood supply: do we need rest, stress, and delayed acquisition? Comparison with SPECT. Radiology 2014;270(3):708–16.

56. Delgado Sanchez-Gracian C, Oca Pernas R, Trinidad Lopez C, et al. Quantitative myocardial perfusion with stress dual-energy CT: iodine concentration differences between normal and ischemic or necrotic myocardium. Initial experience. Eur Radiol 2016;26(9):3199–207.

57. Lu GM, Zhao Y, Zhang LJ, et al. Dual-energy CT of the lung. AJR Am J Roentgenol 2012;199(5 Suppl): S40–53.

58. Zhang LJ, Zhou CS, Schoepf UJ, et al. Dual-energy CT lung ventilation/perfusion imaging for diagnosing pulmonary embolism. Eur Radiol 2013;23(10): 2666–75.

59. Zhang LJ, Lu GM, Meinel FG, et al. Computed tomography of acute pulmonary embolism: state-of-the-art. Eur Radiol 2015;25(9):2547–57.

60. Thieme SF, Becker CR, Hacker M, et al. Dual energy CT for the assessment of lung perfusion—correlation to scintigraphy. Eur J Radiol 2008;68(3):369–74.

61. Okada M, Kunihiro Y, Nakashima Y, et al. Added value of lung perfused blood volume images using dual-energy CT for assessment of acute pulmonary embolism. Eur J Radiol 2015;84(1):172–7.

62. Apfaltrer P, Bachmann V, Meyer M, et al. Prognostic value of perfusion defect volume at dual energy CTA in patients with pulmonary embolism: correlation with CTA obstruction scores, CT parameters of right ventricular dysfunction and adverse clinical outcome. Eur J Radiol 2012;81(11):3592–7.

63. Bauer RW, Frellesen C, Renker M, et al. Dual energy CT pulmonary blood volume assessment in acute pulmonary embolism - correlation with D-dimer level, right heart strain and clinical outcome. Eur Radiol 2011;21(9):1914–21.

64. Meinel FG, Graef A, Bamberg F, et al. Effectiveness of automated quantification of pulmonary perfused blood volume using dual-energy CTPA for the severity assessment of acute pulmonary embolism. Invest Radiol 2013;48(8):563–9.

65. Kong X, Sheng HX, Lu GM, et al. Xenon-enhanced dual-energy CT lung ventilation imaging: techniques and clinical applications. Am J Roentgenol 2014; 202(2):309–17.

66. Ameli-Renani S, Rahman F, Nair A, et al. Dual-energy CT for imaging of pulmonary hypertension: challenges and opportunities. Radiographics 2014; 34(7):1769–90.

67. Dournes G, Verdier D, Montaudon M, et al. Dual-energy CT perfusion and angiography in chronic thromboembolic pulmonary hypertension: diagnostic accuracy and concordance with radionuclide scintigraphy. Eur Radiol 2014;24(1):42–51.

68. Ameli-Renani S, Ramsay L, Bacon JL, et al. Dual-energy computed tomography in the assessment of vascular and parenchymal enhancement in suspected pulmonary hypertension. J Thorac Imaging 2014;29(2):98–106.

69. Obaid DR, Calvert PA, Gopalan D, et al. Dual-energy computed tomography imaging to determine atherosclerotic plaque composition: a prospective study with tissue validation. J Cardiovasc Comput Tomogr 2014;8(3):230–7.

70. Barreto M, Schoenhagen P, Nair A, et al. Potential of dual-energy computed tomography to characterize atherosclerotic plaque: ex vivo assessment of human coronary arteries in comparison to histology. J Cardiovasc Comput Tomogr 2008;2(4):234–42.

71. Tesche C, Caruso D, De Cecco CN, et al. Coronary computed tomography angiography-derived plaque quantification in patients with acute coronary syndrome. Am J Cardiol 2016;119(5):712–8.

72. Tesche C, Plank F, De Cecco CN, et al. Prognostic implications of coronary CT angiography-derived quantitative markers for the prediction of major adverse cardiac events. J Cardiovasc Comput Tomogr 2016;10(6):458–65.

73. Tesche C, De Cecco CN, Vliegenthart R, et al. Coronary CT angiography-derived quantitative markers

for predicting in-stent restenosis. J Cardiovasc Comput Tomogr 2016;10(5):377–83.

74. Henzler T, Porubsky S, Kayed H, et al. Attenuation-based characterization of coronary atherosclerotic plaque: comparison of dual source and dual energy CT with single-source CT and histopathology. Eur J Radiol 2011;80(1):54–9.

75. Ravanfar Haghighi R, Chatterjee S, Tabin M, et al. DECT evaluation of noncalcified coronary artery plaque. Med Phys 2015;42(10):5945–54.

76. Lee H-J, Im DJ, Youn J-C, et al. Myocardial extracellular volume fraction with dual-energy equilibrium contrast-enhanced cardiac CT in nonischemic cardiomyopathy: a prospective comparison with cardiac MR imaging. Radiology 2016;280(1):49–57.

77. Bandula S, White SK, Flett AS, et al. Measurement of myocardial extracellular volume fraction by using equilibrium contrast-enhanced CT: validation against histologic findings. Radiology 2013;269(2):396–403.

78. Hazirolan T, Akpinar B, Ünal S, et al. Value of dual energy computed tomography for detection of myocardial iron deposition in thalassaemia patients: initial experience. Eur J Radiol 2008;68(3):442–5.

Role of Dual-Energy Computed Tomography in Thoracic Oncology

Erika G. Odisio, MD[a], Mylene T. Truong, MD[a],
Cihan Duran, MD[b], Patricia M. de Groot, MD[a],
Myrna C. Godoy, MD, PhD[a],*

KEYWORDS

- Dual-energy CT • Spectral imaging • Pulmonary blood volume • Pulmonary nodule • Lung cancer
- Iodine map • Thoracic malignancy • Virtual noncontrast image

KEY POINTS

- Dual-energy CT (DECT) imaging has broadened the potential of thoracic oncologic imaging by offering multiple postprocessing datasets with a single acquisition.
- The most commonly used material-specific imaging techniques in thoracic oncologic imaging include virtual noncontrast (VNC) imaging, iodine-enhanced image (iodine map), automatic bone removal, and pulmonary blood volume (PBV).
- The characterization of the degree and pattern of contrast enhancement in solitary pulmonary nodules (SPNs) is considered valuable in differentiating benign and malignant nodules with a suggested cutoff value of 20 Hounsfield units of iodine uptake at DECT images acquired 3 minutes after intravenous contrast administration.
- 3-D iodine-related attenuation (IRA), also known as iodine volume, of primary lung cancers is significantly associated with tumor differentiation grade, where high-grade tumors tend to have lower iodine volumes than low-grade tumors. Future directions for the use of DECT include the potential correlation of iodine uptake with gene expression.
- DECT improves characterization of metastatic disease in patients with thoracic malignancies and has potential applications in assessment of tumor response to chemotherapy, radiation therapy planning, and prediction of tumor recurrence.

INTRODUCTION

Dual-energy CT (DECT) imaging has broadened the potential of thoracic oncologic imaging by offering multiple postprocessing datasets with a single acquisition. Although conventional single-energy CT imaging results in an anatomic depiction of the imaged area based on differences in physical density between adjacent structures, DECT imaging extends this capability because, in principle, structures of a similar density but with different elemental compositions may be distinguished based on differing photon absorption at different photon energies.[1] Hence, DECT imaging enhances the physical density anatomic display made possible with single-energy CT by moving toward imaging elemental composition within a given structure. This technique attempts to differentiate specific materials in the generated images, the so-called material specific imaging,

Disclosure Statement: Research Grant Siemens Healthcare (M.C. Godoy).
[a] Department of Diagnostic Radiology, The University of Texas MD Anderson Cancer Center, 1515 Holcombe Boulevard, Houston, TX 77030, USA; [b] Department of Diagnostic Radiology, University of Texas Medical Branch, 301 University Boulevard, Room 2820 JSA, Galveston, TX 77555-0709, USA
* Corresponding author. Department of Diagnostic Radiology, The University of Texas MD Anderson Cancer Center, 1515 Holcombe Boulevard, Unit Number 1478, Houston, TX 77030.
E-mail address: mgodoy@mdanderson.org

Radiol Clin N Am 56 (2018) 535–548
https://doi.org/10.1016/j.rcl.2018.03.011

for example, to selectively depict iodine distribution within an image.[1] Only substances with strong photoelectric effect, however, such as calcium, iodine, barium, and xenon, for example, can be easily differentiated from other body tissues that have weak photoelectric effect.[2]

Current DECT acquisition methods include dual-source scanner with 2 tube-detector systems with or without beam filtration, rapid voltage switching (spectral imaging), dual-layer detector, split filter technique, and sequential scanning. Besides the low and high peak kilovoltage image series, a weighted average image dataset (most similar to conventional 120 kVp images) and virtual monoenergetic or monochromatic image series (VMIs) are usually reconstructed for clinical interpretation. In addition, several material-specific imaging applications are currently available. The most commonly used material-specific imaging techniques in thoracic imaging include virtual noncontrast (VNC) imaging, iodine-enhanced image (iodine map), automatic bone removal, and pulmonary blood volume (PBV). The use of these techniques has shown established advantages and promising new directions for thoracic oncologic imaging, including evaluation of lung nodules and thoracic malignancies, staging of lung cancer, surgical planning, assessment of response to treatment, and characterization of complications, such as incidental pulmonary embolism (PE). The purpose of this article is to review the current status of clinical applications for DECT in thoracic oncology.

INDETERMINATE SOLITARY PULMONARY NODULE AND LUNG MASSES

DECT permits quantification of the degree of enhancement and identification of calcification of the lung nodules in a single postcontrast CT acquisition without the need of precontrast image acquisition, therefore lowering radiation dose.[3]

The characterization of the degree and pattern of contrast enhancement in SPNs is considered valuable in differentiating benign and malignant nodules. A study of Chae and colleagues[3] evaluated 49 patients with pulmonary nodules scanned before and 3 minutes after intravenous contrast administration. They compared CT numbers of SPN on true nonenhanced weighted average images and VNC images as well as the CT number of SPN on iodine-enhanced image (iodine map) and the actual degree of enhancement (CT number on enhanced weighted average image minus CT number on nonenhanced weighted average image), showing good correlation. The diagnostic accuracy for characterization of malignant nodules using a cutoff value of 20 Hounsfield units (HU) of iodine uptake on iodine-enhanced image was comparable to that of using the degree of enhancement (sensitivity, 92% and 72%; specificity, 70% and 70%; and accuracy, 82.2% and 71.1%), highlighting the potential of DECT to improve SPN characterization in a single postcontrast acquisition without additional radiation dose (Fig. 1).[3] On VNC images, 85.0% (17 of 20) of calcifications in the SPN and 97.8% (44 of 45) of

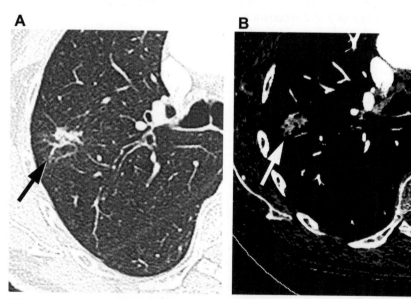

Fig. 1. SPN. (*A*) Lung window settings image shows an irregular right upper lobe nodule (*arrow*). (*B*) Color-coded Iodine map image shows contrast enhancement (35 HU of iodine uptake) (*arrow*). Biopsy reveled lung adenocarcinoma. A threshold of 20 HU of iodine uptake at DECT acquired 3 min after intravenous contrast administration has been proposed to differentiate benign from malignant lung nodules.

calcifications in the lymph nodes were detected, although the apparent sizes were smaller than those on the nonenhanced weighted average images.[3]

The use of DECT in the evaluation of pulmonary ground-glass nodules (GGNs) has been subject of study recently. Kawai and colleagues[4] showed that DECT was able to detect and quantify iodine concentration in a GGN phantom model as well as in GGNs from 24 patients. The contrast enhancement was visible in 22 adenocarcinomas but not in pulmonary hemorrhage and inflammatory changes.[4]

The value of DECT in the differentiation of lung cancer from inflammatory masses using quantitative net enhancement measured on 70 keV monochromatic images has also been demonstrated. In a study by Hou and colleagues,[5] despite similar peak enhancement value in malignant and inflammatory masses, the DECT-derived iodine concentration in the central region of inflammatory lung masses was higher than that of lung cancers. The slopes of spectral attenuation curves at central and peripheral regions of the mass were also higher in inflammatory lesions. Differences in iodine net enhancement between central and peripheral regions of the mass indicated higher heterogeneity in lung cancers, as opposed to the high and homogeneous enhancement of inflammatory lesions.

Lung Cancer

More recently, the role of DECT for characterization of tumor invasiveness has been evaluated. A prospective study by Son and colleagues[6] evaluated 39 subsolid nodules that underwent DECT followed by complete tumor resection, which included 4 adenocarcinomas in situ (10%), 9 minimally invasive adenocarcinomas (23%), and 26 invasive adenocarcinomas (67%). When assessing only VNC imaging, multivariate analysis revealed that mass, uniformity, and size-zone variability were independent predictors of invasive adenocarcinoma (odds ratio [OR] = 19.92, $P = .02$; OR = 0.70, $P = .01$; and OR = 16.16, $P = .04$, respectively). After assessing iodine-enhanced imaging with VNC imaging, the parameters of mass on the VNC imaging and uniformity on the iodine-enhanced imaging were independent predictors of invasive adenocarcinoma (OR = 5.51, $P = .04$, and OR = 0.67, $P<.01$), showing that the addition of the iodine-enhanced imaging parameters (heterogeneity of the enhancement of the GGNs) improved detection of invasive adenocarcinoma versus VNC imaging alone.[6]

Another study with 63 non–small cell lung cancer (NSCLC) lesions by Shimamoto and colleagues[7] demonstrated that 3-D iodine-related attenuation (3D-IRA), also known as iodine volume, of primary lung cancers measured by DECT was significantly associated with their differentiation grade, where high-grade tumors tended to have lower iodine volumes than low-grade tumors. The mean attenuation ±SD of the 3D-IRA was 56.1 HU ± 22.6 HU in well-differentiated tumors, 48.5 HU ± 23.9 HU in moderately differentiated tumors, and 28.4 HU ± 15.8 HU in poorly differentiated tumors. In addition they reported that low 3D-IRA tumors tend to have greater invasiveness that high 3D-IRA tumors. In this study, multivariate logistic analysis revealed that only the corrected 3D-IRA was significantly correlated with tumor invasiveness ($P = .003$), whereas gender, clinical size, and solid/subsolid type were not ($P = .950$, $P = .057$, and $P = .456$, respectively) (**Fig. 2**).[7]

Future directions for the use of DECT comprise the potential correlation of iodine uptake with gene expression. A recent study by Yanagawa and colleagues[8] included 18 patients with adenocarcinoma of the lung who underwent DE dynamic multiphase CT. The study of solitary lung nodules (6 part-solid and 12 solid nodules) showed that iodine content at 2-minute and 3-minute delayed scan might correlate with the expression level of hypoxia-inducible factor 1α.[8] Correlation between the expression level of vascular endothelial growth factor in NSCLC tissue as a biomarker for tumor angiogenesis and the quantitative parameters of spectral CT imaging has also been demonstrated by Li and colleagues.[9] In this study that evaluated 48 cases of NSCLC, the parameters of iodine concentrations, the slope of the spectral HU curve (λHU) values, and CT values at 40 keV all displayed a significant and positive correlation with the level of vascular endothelial growth factor expression (r = 0.413, r = 0.458, and r = 0.393, respectively; $P<.05$).[9]

MEDIASTINAL LYMPH NODES

DECT may assist in characterization of metastatic nodal involvement in cancer staging. In this regard, Tawfik and colleagues[10] have demonstrated that DECT derived iodine content differs significantly between normal, inflammatory, and metastatic squamous cell carcinoma in cervical lymph nodes. Similarly, Li and colleagues[11] demonstrated that DECT iodine concentration can be used to differentiate metastatic from benign lymph nodes in patients with NSCLC. In their study, thresholds of 29.32 100 mg/cm^3 for iodine concentration and

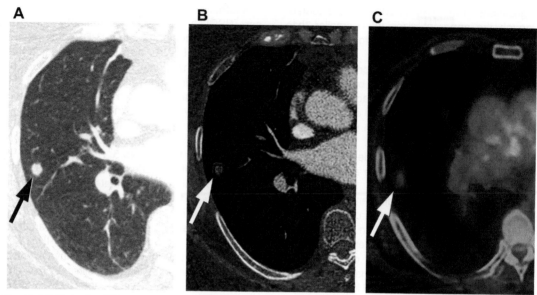

Fig. 2. Moderately differentiated lung adenocarcinoma. (*A*) Lung window settings image shows a well-circumscribed right middle lobe nodule (*arrow*). (*B*) 100/Sn140 kVp image with color-coded iodine map overlay shows iodine uptake (*arrow*). Lung nodule application software showed 3D-IRA of 34 HU. (*C*) Fused PET/CT image demonstrates FDG avidity (SUVmax 3.8) (*arrow*). 3D-IRA is associated with the degree of differentiation in primary lung cancers. Good correlation has been demonstrated between iodine uptake on DECT and metabolic activity on PET/CT.

0.43 for normalized iodine concentration were suggested to detect nodal metastasis with 80% and 75% sensitivity; 70% and 75% specificity; 70% and 75% positive predictive value; 76% and 75% negative predictive value; 73% and 75% accuracy, respectively. In another study by Yang and colleagues[12] that evaluated a total of 144 lymph nodes, including 48 metastatic lymph nodes and 96 non-metastatic lymph nodes, the λHU measured during both arterial and venous phases were significantly higher in metastatic than in benign lymph nodes ($P<.05$). The area under the receiver operating characteristic curve (AUC = 0.951) of λHU of the arterial phase was the largest. Using 2.75 as the optimal threshold value of λHU, the sensitivity, specificity, and overall accuracy in the diagnosis of metastatic lymph nodes were 88.2%, 88.4%, and 87.0%, respectively.[12]

The use of fluorine-18-fluorodeoxyglucose (FDG) PET/CT has become standard of care in lung cancer staging in the United States. A study by Schmid-Bindert and colleagues[13] demonstrated a strong correlation between PET/CT maximum standardized uptake value (SUVmax) and DECT IRA (interval of <21 days between DECT and PET/CT) in thoracic metastatic lymph nodes (r = 0.654, $P = .010$) as well as in the primary malignancy (r = 0.768, $P = .017$, and n = 17 patients), suggesting that DECT could serve as a valuable functional imaging test.

MEDIASTINAL MASSES, PERICARDIUM, HEART, AND PLEURA

There are few data available on the role of DECT in the characterization of other thoracic malignancies. Because angiogenesis is a fundamental process in the development of tumors, iodine concentration measurements with DECT data provide a reliable quantitative parameter to indicate lesion enhancement, which could help radiologists differentiate between benign and malignant lesions in the mediastinum, heart, pericardium, and pleura. In addition, availability of VNC images may add information in characterization of thoracic lesions, such as in the differentiation between enhancing pleural lesions versus pleurodesis (**Fig. 3**).

It has been shown that iodine overlay images can be used to successfully differentiate benign and malignant mediastinal tumors. Lee and colleagues[14] evaluated 25 patients with suspected mediastinal tumors and found that the iodine concentration measurements were significantly different between benign and malignant tumors both in the early phase (1.38 mg/mL vs 2.41 mg/mL, $P = .001$) and in the delayed phase (1.52 mg/mL vs 2.84 mg/mL, $P = .001$), whereas traditional mean attenuation values were not significantly different in the 2 phases (57.8 HU vs 69.1 HU; $P = .067$; and 67.4 HU vs 78.4 HU, $P = .086$, respectively).

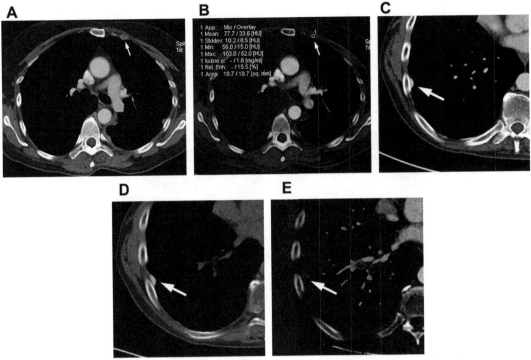

Fig. 3. DECT characterization of pleural lesions. (A) 100/Sn140 image reveals a lesion in the left anterior hemithorax (arrow), concerning for pleural metastases in a patient with lung adenocarcinoma. (B) Iodine map overlay demonstrates iodine uptake of 33.6 HU (arrow). Increase in size during short-term follow-up CT confirmed malignancy. (C) 100/Sn140 kVp image shows a high attenuation pleural lesion in a different patient (arrow). This finding could mimic an enhancing pleural lesion. However, VNC image (D) demonstrates high attenuation not related to iodine contrast (arrow). (E) Iodine map overlay image confirms lack of iodine uptake (arrow). Clinical correlation confirmed history of talc pleurodesis.

Another potential application of quantitative analysis in DECT is the differentiation between intracardiac or pulmonary artery thrombus and tumor. Chang and colleagues[15] evaluated filling defects in the main pulmonary artery on DECT of 19 patients, including 6 patients with pulmonary artery sarcoma (PAS) and 13 with pulmonary thromboembolism (PTE). The mean HU values were not significantly different between the PTE and PAS groups (45.5 ± 15.9 vs 47.1 ± 9.2 HU; $P = .776$). The mean IRA and iodine concentration values of the lesions were significantly different, however, between the PTE and PAS groups (10.6 ± 7.2 vs 27.9 ± 9.1 HU, $P = .004$; and 0.61 ± 0.39 vs 1.49 ± 0.57, $P = .001$).

METASTATIC DISEASE TO THE LIVER AND ADRENAL GLANDS

DECT improves characterization of metastatic disease in patients with thoracic malignancies. It has been shown that DECT-derived low peak kilovoltage imaging demonstrates greater attenuation differences between metastatic liver disease and normal hepatic parenchyma and a better contrast-to-noise ratio (CNR) than conventional 120-kVp single-energy CT data, improving the conspicuity of even subtle metastatic lesions (Fig. 4).[16,17] The same differences for these data sets are found for hypervascular hepatic lesions during the late arterial phase of enhancement.[18]

VNC images may allow the characterization of incidental adrenal masses with good accuracy compared with standard single energy CT nonenhanced images, particularly for incidental adrenal masses at least 1 cm in diameter, and therefore have potential to replace unenhanced images (Fig. 5).[19] In addition, a decrease in attenuation of an adrenal lesion between 140 kVp and 80 kVp is a highly specific sign of adrenal adenoma as an indicator of intracellular lipid.[20] In a study that evaluated 31 adrenal nodules including 26 adenomas and 5 metastatic nodules, the mean attenuation change between 140 kVp and 80 kVp was 0.4 HU ± 7.1 HU for adenomas and 9.2 HU ± 4.3 HU for metastatic lesions ($P<.003$); 50% of adenomas had an attenuation decrease at 80 kVp and all metastatic lesions had an

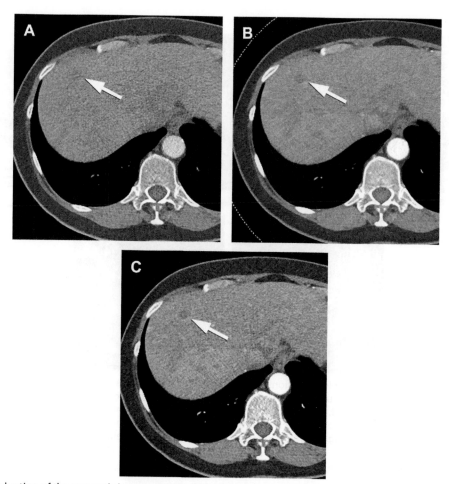

Fig. 4. Evaluation of the upper abdomen on a chest CT of a patient with lung cancer. (*A*) Sn140 kVp, (*B*) 100/Sn140 weighted average and (*C*) 80 kVp images. Note improved conspicuity of a subtle metastatic liver lesion (*arrows*) at low kilovoltage imaging (*C*). When compared with 120 kVp data, 80 kVp data acquired from DECT has been proven to demonstrate greater attenuation differences and improved contrast to noise between metastatic disease and normal liver.

attenuation increase at 80 kVp. With a decrease in attenuation at 80 kVp as an indicator of intracellular lipid within an adenoma, DECT has 50% sensitivity, 100% specificity, 100% positive predictive value, and 28% negative predictive value in the diagnosis of adenoma.[20] Another study by Shi and colleagues[21] evaluated the mean attenuation value changes (MAVCs) between 140 kVp and 80 kVp (MAVC140 kVp–MAVC80 kVp) as well as the MAVCx between 100 keV and 40 keV (MAVC100–MAVC40 keV) in 63 adrenal nodules. When the cutoff points were set at 2.42 HU and 6.95 HU for MAVC140 kVp to MAVC80 kVp and MAVC100 keV to MAVC40 keV, the 2 parameters both had a sensitivity of 78.6% and a specificity of 100% in adenoma diagnosis.[21] According to these studies, the unique energy spectrum information provided by DECT shows high capacity to distinguish adrenal adenoma from metastasis.

ONCOLOGIC SURGICAL PLANNING

The evaluation of tumor size and invasion to adjacent structures can be optimized with multiplanar reconstructions, three-dimensional volume rendering and bone removal application for surgical planning (**Fig. 6**). DECT derived low-energy imaging improves iodine contrast opacification and, therefore, allows better characterization of vascular structures, which permits the evaluation of possible vascular involvement by tumors and primary vascular pathologies that may affect surgical management.[22,23] In addition, the prediction of postoperative lung function in patients undergoing lung resection is important because poor respiratory function in patients with resectable lung cancer may interfere with surgical treatment due to increased risk for perioperative morbidity, mortality, and postoperative long-term disability. A study

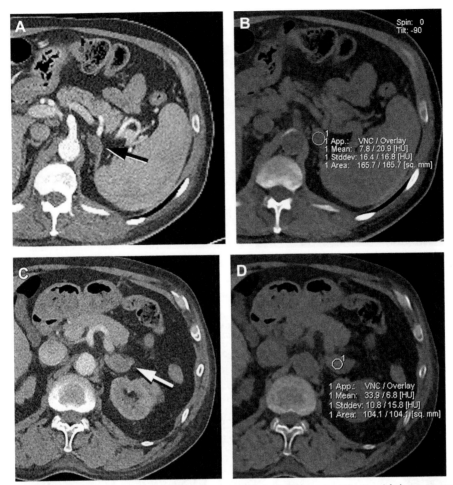

Fig. 5. (*A, B*) Adrenal adenoma and (*C, D*) adrenal metastasis in 2 different patients with lung cancer (*arrows*). VNC images show lower attenuation of the adenoma on VNC imaging (*B*, 7.8 HU) compared with the metastatic lesion (*D*, 33.9 HU). Diagnosis was confirmed by MRI and imaging follow-up. VNC images have potential to replace unenhanced images for characterization of adrenal lesions seen in patients with thoracic malignancy.

by Chae and colleagues[24] evaluated 51 patients with lung cancer undergoing lung resection and compared the use of DECT PBV versus the standard use of perfusion scintigraphy for prediction of postoperative lung function. Lobe segmentation and lobar perfusion ratio were performed using a software developed in-house. Their group reported a 15.4% versus 17.8% error in postoperative estimation of forced expiratory volume in the first second of expiration with DECT versus scintigraphy, respectively, suggesting that DECT may have a higher accuracy.[24] Compared with perfusion scintigraphy, DECT has higher spatial resolution for the assessment of the lobe to be resected and greater accuracy for calculation of both the regional and total lung volumes. Upon validation of this technique in a larger cohort with commercially available software, DECT has potential to replace lung perfusion scintigraphy using inherent

information obtained from CT images acquired for tumor staging, therefore decreasing radiation exposure and cost.

RADIATION THERAPY

Although current clinical evidence for the use of DECT in radiation therapy is still limited, multiple potential applications have been identified in this field, including improvements in radiation therapy planning with more precise dose calculation and metal artifact reduction as well as improved tumor delineation and normal tissue characterization (**Fig. 7**).[25,26]

Integration of functional information in lung radiation therapy planning has the potential to spare the most functional lung areas. Use of single-photon emission CT (SPECT)/CT– derived function has previously been extensively described in lung radiation therapy. A small study by Lapointe and

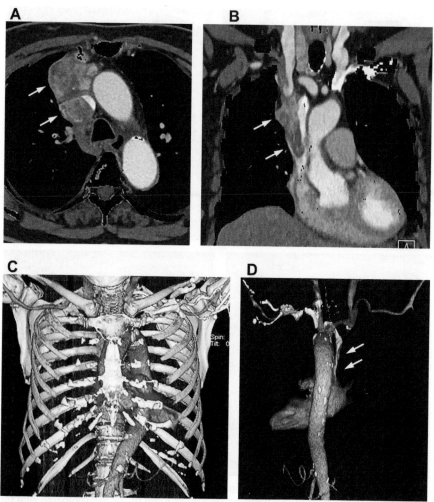

Fig. 6. DECT bone removal application. (*A*) Axial and (*B*) coronal images with bone removal, (*C*) 3D volume rendering (VR), and (*D*) rotated 3D-VR image with bone removal of a patient with invasive thymoma and SVC invasion (*arrows*). 3D-VR images helps to evaluate the extension of disease and DECT bone removal application decreases 3D-VR reconstruction time.

colleagues[27] showed good agreement between iodine concentration maps from DECT and SPECT/CT for the assessment of lung volumes or function, highlighting the potential of the use of DECT to spare functional lung tissues during radiation therapy. Similarly, a study that evaluated 25 patients with lung cancer undergoing stereotactic ablative radiation therapy for early-stage disease or intensity modulated radiation therapy for locally advanced disease showed that lobar function derived from a DECT iodine map correlates well with SPECT/CT, and its integration in lung treatment planning is associated with significant differences in the percent lung volume receiving 5 Gy (V5) and mean lung dose to anatomic versus functional lungs.[25]

The prognostic impact of DECT-derived iodine concentration in lung tumors treated with stereotactic body radiotherapy has also been investigated. Aoki and colleagues[28] reported that iodine uptake at the arterial phase of DECT is a useful biomarker for predicting lung cancer recurrence after stereotactic body radiotherapy. That is, tumors with lower iodine uptake at pretreatment evaluation showed worse prognosis after radiotherapy, presumably indicating radio-resistance in hypoxic cell populations in tumors.

The potential use of DECT to improve accuracy in the detection of tumor recurrence after radiation therapy has yet to be investigated (**Figs. 8** and **9**).

CHEMOTHERAPY

DECT has potential to improve the assessment of tumor response to chemotherapy (**Fig. 10**). Kim and colleagues[29] have demonstrated that the

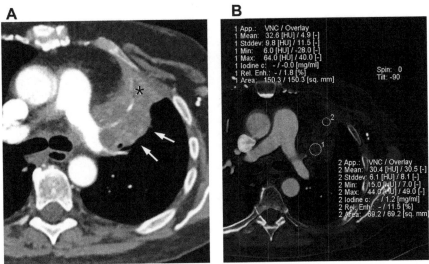

Fig. 7. DECT in radiation therapy planning for lung cancer. (*A*) 100/Sn140kVp weighted average and (*B*) VNC with iodine map overlay images. Left upper lobe central mass (*arrows*) and post obstructive atelectasis (*asterisk*) could be better differentiated with color-coded iodine map (*B*). Note 30 HU of iodine uptake in the atelectatic lung versus 4.9 HU in the central mass. Improved tumor delineation contributes to radiotherapy therapy planning.

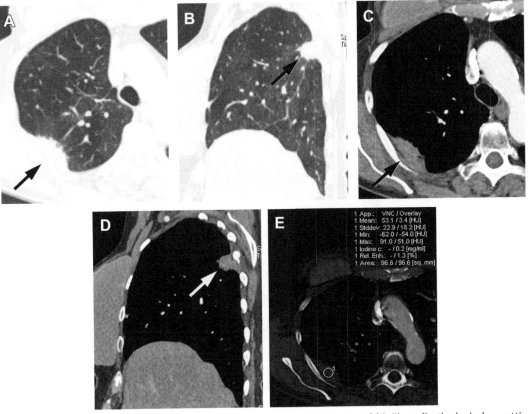

Fig. 8. DECT evaluation after radiation therapy for lung cancer. (*A, B*) Lung and (*C, D*) mediastinal window setting images show a spiculated mass in the right upper lobe (*arrows*) suspicious for tumor recurrence after radiation therapy. (*E*) VNC with iodine map overlay image shows only 3.4 HU of iodine uptake suggesting benign etiology. Biopsy revealed no viable tumor.

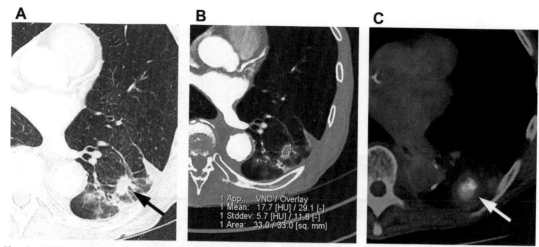

Fig. 9. DECT evaluation after radiation therapy for lung cancer. (*A*) Lung window setting image shows a left lower lobe nodule within the radiation field consistent with the treated malignancy (*arrow*). (*B*) VNC with iodine map overlay image shows 29 HU of iodine uptake within the nodule. (*C*) PET/CT fused image shows high FDG uptake (SUVmax 8) suspicious for residual or recurrent tumor (*arrow*). Fine-needle aspiration revealed viable squamous cell carcinoma.

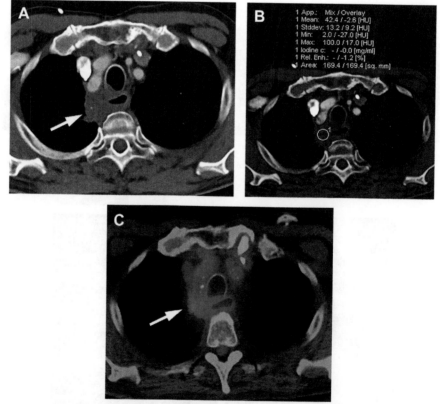

Fig. 10. Assessment of response to concurrent chemoradiation therapy in a patient with squamous cell carcinoma. A persistent right upper lobe paramediastinal soft tissue mass (*arrows*) raised concern for residual viable tumor. (*A*) 100/Sn140 and (*B*) iodine map overly images show low level of iodine enhancement in the tumor (2.6 HU), suggesting response to the therapy. (*C*) PET/CT image shows concordant low FDG uptake (SUV max 3.5, previously 20.3 before treatment). Biopsy showed absence of viable tumor.

quantification of iodine net enhancement may serve as a useful tool for assessing tumor response to treatment with antiangiogenic agents in patients with NSCLC and that VNC images could distinguish intratumor hemorrhage from tumor enhancement in these patients, avoiding misinterpretation of progressive disease in cases with hemorrhage causing increase in tumor size. Their study showed 16% discordance between tumor response in target lesions based on Response Evaluation Criteria in Solid Tumors version 1.1 versus response assessment using a modified Choi's criteria with DECT, which takes into account not only changes in tumor size but also iodine net enhancement.[29–31]

More recently, Baxa and colleagues[32] reported that iodine uptake quantification in dual-phase DECT shows potential benefit in assessment of anti-EGFR therapy response. They demonstrated a decrease in vascularization in the responding primary tumors and nonsignificant variable development of vascularization in nonresponding tumors. A significant difference of percentage change in the arterial enhancement fraction (ratio of iodine uptake in the arterial and venous phase) was reported between responders and nonresponders (P = .019–.043).

The use of DECT quantitative parameters is a promising tool for the evaluation of the primary malignancy as well as therapy response in metastatic lymph nodes. In a study for the assessment of lymph node staging and therapy response in 27 patients with lung cancer, there was a significant decrease in enhancement in responding metastatic lymph nodes when comparing dual-energy data of prechemotherapy and post chemotherapy CT studies.[33]

PULMONARY EMBOLISM

PE is a frequent cause of morbidity and mortality in oncologic patients, sometimes detected incidentally in this patient population.[34] In cases of suboptimal contrast opacification of the pulmonary arteries, low-energy monochromatic images (50 keV–70 keV) can be assessed to increase the confidence for the diagnosis of PE compared with conventional single-energy CT given increased contrast attenuation at low-energy imaging.[35–37] Recently, the introduction of the advanced VMI reconstruction algorithm (monoplus) further improved CNR in DECT imaging based on the association of high contrast from low-kilovoltage data set with low noise of high-kilovoltage data set from VMI (nonlinear blending).[38] In a study by Meier and colleagues,[38] the use of monoplus images at 40 keV showed significant improvement of contrast conspicuity compared with 60 keV conventional VMI imaging for the analysis of CT pulmonary angiography.

Given the higher attenuation of iodine at lower energy levels, DECT allows CT pulmonary angiography to be performed with contrast media dose reduction of up to one-third of the standard amount while still maintaining adequate image quality for PE evaluation.[35,36,38,39] This benefit is especially relevant for oncologic patients with multiple comorbidities, potentially undergoing nephrotoxic therapy, who undergo multiple CT scans during the course of their treatment.

In addition to the improved characterization of endoluminal filling defects due to increased contrast attenuation at DECT low-energy imaging, the use of the DECT PBV application can add functional information regarding lung perfusion.[40] The PBV application displays the iodine distribution in each voxel of the lung parenchyma at a single time point after the administration of intravenous contrast material and can be used as a surrogate for lung perfusion with no additional radiation exposure.[1,24,41–43] PBV allows the evaluation of lung perfusion defects caused by emboli with good agreement with ventilation/perfusion scintigraphy and adds functional information that may help differentiate occlusive from nonocclusive PE, once complete arterial obstruction is necessary to determine perfusion defects.[42,44–47] Pulmonary perfusion defect scoring based on DECT PBV has the potential to serve as an extra or alternative tool in PE severity assessment.[48] In addition, the correlation of PBV images with conventional lung window setting images allows the differential diagnosis for iodine distribution defects.[40] For instance, in the presence of pulmonary infarction, a peripheral wedge-shaped area of "perfusion defect" is seen at PBV images which correlates with the wedge-shaped lung consolidation visualized on lung window settings. On the other hand, decreased "lung perfusion" on PBV images without associated opacities in the lung parenchyma are findings of pulmonary occlusive vascular disease without infarction (**Fig. 11**).[40]

RADIATION DOSE

Evidence suggests that DECT is not associated with an increase in radiation dose comparing with single-source CT, although radiation dose data for rapid kilovoltage switching can be higher than for single-energy CT.[40] Similar radiation doses were found when comparing DECT, single-energy multidetector CT, and dual-source CT without the use of the dual-energy mode.[3] Importantly, the radiation dose from DECT

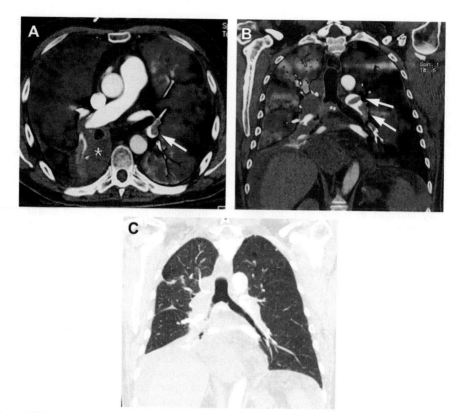

Fig. 11. Lung PBV analysis as a surrogate for lung perfusion. (*A*) Axial and (*B*) coronal 100/Sn140kVp with PBV overlay images show detection of endovascular thrombi (*arrows*) with corresponding wedge-shaped perfusion defects in the left lung in a patient with right lower lobe squamous cell carcinoma (*asterisk*). (*C*) Coronal image with lung window settings shows lack of matching lung opacities demonstrating absence of lung infarct despite the perfusion defect. PE is a common complication in oncologic patients. DECT can identify perfusion defects caused by occlusive thrombi and can differentiate perfusion defects with or without pulmonary infarcts.

depends on specific parameters, such as tube current, pitch, and energy. For instance, dual-energy images may be obtained at radiation doses similar to those of single-energy images if low tube currents are used.[16] For imaging protocols in which true unenhanced images could be replaced with VNC images, the radiation dose from DECT may be reduced.[16,49]

SUMMARY

DECT is an emerging technology that has potential to enhance diagnostic performance and radiologists' confidence in the evaluation of thoracic malignancies. DECT clinical applications include characterization of SPN, lung masses, and mediastinal tumors. DECT–derived iodine uptake quantification may assist in characterization of tumor differentiation and gene expression. The use DECT in oncology has potential to improve lung cancer staging, therapy planning, and assessment of response to therapy as well as detection of incidental PE.

ACKNOWLEDGMENTS

The authors thank the support provided by the John S. Dunn, Sr. Distinguished Chair in Diagnostic Imaging.

REFERENCES

1. Godoy MC, Naidich DP, Marchiori E, et al. Basic principles and postprocessing techniques of dual-energy CT: illustrated by selected congenital abnormalities of the thorax. J Thorac Imaging 2009;24(2):152–9.
2. Goo HW, Goo JM. Dual-energy CT: new horizon in medical imaging. Korean J Radiol 2017;18(4):555–69.
3. Chae EJ, Song JW, Seo JB, et al. Clinical utility of dual-energy CT in the evaluation of solitary pulmonary nodules: initial experience. Radiology 2008; 249(2):671–81.
4. Kawai T, Shibamoto Y, Hara M, et al. Can dual-energy CT evaluate contrast enhancement of ground-glass attenuation? Phantom and preliminary clinical studies. Acad Radiol 2011;18(6):682–9.
5. Hou WS, Wu HW, Yin Y, et al. Differentiation of lung cancers from inflammatory masses with dual-

energy spectral CT imaging. Acad Radiol 2015; 22(3):337–44.

6. Son JY, Lee HY, Kim JH, et al. Quantitative CT analysis of pulmonary ground-glass opacity nodules for distinguishing invasive adenocarcinoma from non-invasive or minimally invasive adenocarcinoma: the added value of using iodine mapping. Eur Radiol 2016;26(1):43–54.

7. Shimamoto H, Iwano S, Umakoshi H, et al. Evaluation of locoregional invasiveness of small-sized non-small cell lung cancers by enhanced dual-energy computed tomography. Cancer Imaging 2016;16(1):18.

8. Yanagawa M, Morii E, Hata A, et al. Dual-energy dynamic CT of lung adenocarcinoma: correlation of iodine uptake with tumor gene expression. Eur J Radiol 2016;85(8):1407–13.

9. Li GJ, Gao J, Wang GL, et al. Correlation between vascular endothelial growth factor and quantitative dual-energy spectral CT in non-small-cell lung cancer. Clin Radiol 2016;71(4):363–8.

10. Tawfik AM, Razek AA, Kerl JM, et al. Comparison of dual-energy CT-derived iodine content and iodine overlay of normal, inflammatory and metastatic squamous cell carcinoma cervical lymph nodes. Eur Radiol 2014;24(3):574–80.

11. Li X, Meng X, Ye Z. Iodine quantification to characterize primary lesions, metastatic and non-metastatic lymph nodes in lung cancers by dual energy computed tomography: An initial experience. Eur J Radiol 2016;85(6):1219–23.

12. Yang F, Dong J, Wang X, et al. Non-small cell lung cancer: spectral computed tomography quantitative parameters for preoperative diagnosis of metastatic lymph nodes. Eur J Radiol 2017;89:129–35.

13. Schmid-Bindert G, Henzler T, Chu TQ, et al. Functional imaging of lung cancer using dual energy CT: how does iodine related attenuation correlate with standardized uptake value of 18FDG-PET-CT? Eur Radiol 2012;22(1):93–103.

14. Lee SH, Hur J, Kim YJ, et al. Additional value of dual-energy CT to differentiate between benign and malignant mediastinal tumors: an initial experience. Eur J Radiol 2013;82(11):2043–9.

15. Chang S, Hur J, Im DJ, et al. Dual-energy CT-based iodine quantification for differentiating pulmonary artery sarcoma from pulmonary thromboembolism: a pilot study. Eur Radiol 2016;26(9):3162–70.

16. Coursey CA, Nelson RC, Boll DT, et al. Dual-energy multidetector CT: how does it work, what can it tell us, and when can we use it in abdominopelvic imaging? Radiographics 2010;30(4):1037–55.

17. Robinson E, Babb J, Chandarana H, et al. Dual source dual energy MDCT: comparison of 80 kVp and weighted average 120 kVp data for conspicuity of hypo-vascular liver metastases. Invest Radiol 2010;45(7):413–8.

18. Marin D, Boll DT, Mileto A, et al. State of the art: dual-energy CT of the abdomen. Radiology 2014;271(2):327–42.

19. Gnannt R, Fischer M, Goetti R, et al. Dual-energy CT for characterization of the incidental adrenal mass: preliminary observations. AJR Am J Roentgenol 2012;198(1):138–44.

20. Gupta RT, Ho LM, Marin D, et al. Dual-energy CT for characterization of adrenal nodules: initial experience. AJR Am J Roentgenol 2010;194(6):1479–83.

21. Shi JW, Dai HZ, Shen L, et al. Dual-energy CT: clinical application in differentiating an adrenal adenoma from a metastasis. Acta Radiol 2014;55(4):505–12.

22. Ko JP, Brandman S, Stember J, et al. Dual-energy computed tomography: concepts, performance, and thoracic applications. J Thorac Imaging 2012;27(1):7–22.

23. Vlahos I, Godoy MC, Naidich DP. Dual-energy computed tomography imaging of the aorta. J Thorac Imaging 2010;25(4):289–300.

24. Chae EJ, Kim N, Seo JB, et al. Prediction of postoperative lung function in patients undergoing lung resection: dual-energy perfusion computed tomography versus perfusion scintigraphy. Invest Radiol 2013;48(8):622–7.

25. Bahig H, Campeau MP, Lapointe A, et al. Phase 1-2 study of dual-energy computed tomography for assessment of pulmonary function in radiation therapy planning. Int J Radiat Oncol Biol Phys 2017;99(2):334–43.

26. Landry G, Gaudreault M, van Elmpt W, et al. Improved dose calculation accuracy for low energy brachytherapy by optimizing dual energy CT imaging protocols for noise reduction using sinogram affirmed iterative reconstruction. Z Med Phys 2016;26(1):75–87.

27. Lapointe A, Bahig H, Blais D, et al. Assessing lung function using contrast-enhanced dual energy computed tomography for potential applications in radiation therapy. Med Phys 2017;44(10):5260–9.

28. Aoki M, Hirose K, Sato M, et al. Prognostic impact of average iodine density assessed by dual-energy spectral imaging for predicting lung tumor recurrence after stereotactic body radiotherapy. J Radiat Res 2016;57(4):381–6.

29. Kim YN, Lee HY, Lee KS, et al. Dual-energy CT in patients treated with anti-angiogenic agents for non-small cell lung cancer: new method of monitoring tumor response? Korean J Radiol 2012;13(6):702–10.

30. Choi H, Charnsangavej C, Faria SC, et al. Correlation of computed tomography and positron emission tomography in patients with metastatic gastrointestinal stromal tumor treated at a single institution with imatinib mesylate: proposal of new computed

tomography response criteria. J Clin Oncol 2007; 25(13):1753–9.

31. Eisenhauer EA, Therasse P, Bogaerts J, et al. New response evaluation criteria in solid tumours: revised RECIST guideline (version 1.1). Eur J Cancer 2009; 45(2):228–47.

32. Baxa J, Matouskova T, Krakorova G, et al. Dual-phase dual-energy CT in patients treated with erlotinib for advanced non-small cell lung cancer: possible benefits of iodine quantification in response assessment. Eur Radiol 2016;26(8):2828–36.

33. Baxa J, Vondrakova A, Matouskova T, et al. Dual-phase dual-energy CT in patients with lung cancer: assessment of the additional value of iodine quantification in lymph node therapy response. Eur Radiol 2014;24(8):1981–8.

34. Bach AG, Schmoll HJ, Beckel C, et al. Pulmonary embolism in oncologic patients: frequency and embolus burden of symptomatic and unsuspected events. Acta Radiol 2014;55(1):45–53.

35. Delesalle MA, Pontana F, Duhamel A, et al. Spectral optimization of chest CT angiography with reduced iodine load: experience in 80 patients evaluated with dual-source, dual-energy CT. Radiology 2013; 267(1):256–66.

36. Apfaltrer P, Sudarski S, Schneider D, et al. Value of monoenergetic low-kV dual energy CT datasets for improved image quality of CT pulmonary angiography. Eur J Radiol 2014;83(2):322–8.

37. Yuan R, Shuman WP, Earls JP, et al. Reduced iodine load at CT pulmonary angiography with dual-energy monochromatic imaging: comparison with standard CT pulmonary angiography–a prospective randomized trial. Radiology 2012;262(1):290–7.

38. Meier A, Wurnig M, Desbiolles L, et al. Advanced virtual monoenergetic images: improving the contrast of dual-energy CT pulmonary angiography. Clin Radiol 2015;70(11):1244–51.

39. Godoy MC, Heller SL, Naidich DP, et al. Dual-energy MDCT: comparison of pulmonary artery enhancement on dedicated CT pulmonary angiography, routine and low contrast volume studies. Eur J Radiol 2011;79(2):e11–7.

40. Otrakji A, Digumarthy SR, Lo Gullo R, et al. Dual-energy CT: spectrum of thoracic abnormalities. Radiographics 2016;36(1):38–52.

41. Kim BH, Seo JB, Chae EJ, et al. Analysis of perfusion defects by causes other than acute pulmonary thromboembolism on contrast-enhanced dual-energy CT in consecutive 537 patients. Eur J Radiol 2012;81(4):e647–652.

42. Hagspiel KD, Flors L, Housseini AM, et al. Pulmonary blood volume imaging with dual-energy computed tomography: spectrum of findings. Clin Radiol 2012;67(1):69–77.

43. Pontana F, Remy-Jardin M, Duhamel A, et al. Lung perfusion with dual-energy multi-detector row CT: can it help recognize ground glass opacities of vascular origin? Acad Radiol 2010;17(5): 587–94.

44. Thieme SF, Becker CR, Hacker M, et al. Dual energy CT for the assessment of lung perfusion–correlation to scintigraphy. Eur J Radiol 2008; 68(3):369–74.

45. Thieme SF, Johnson TR, Lee C, et al. Dual-energy CT for the assessment of contrast material distribution in the pulmonary parenchyma. AJR Am J Roentgenol 2009;193(1):144–9.

46. Meinel FG, Graef A, Bamberg F, et al. Effectiveness of automated quantification of pulmonary perfused blood volume using dual-energy CTPA for the severity assessment of acute pulmonary embolism. Invest Radiol 2013;48(8):563–9.

47. Remy-Jardin M, Faivre JB, Pontana F, et al. Thoracic applications of dual energy. Semin Respir Crit Care Med 2014;35(1):64–73.

48. Thieme SF, Ashoori N, Bamberg F, et al. Severity assessment of pulmonary embolism using dual energy CT- correlation of a pulmonary perfusion defect score with clinical and morphological parameters of blood oxygenation and right ventricular failure. Eur Radiol 2012;22(2):269–78.

49. Chandarana H, Godoy MC, Vlahos I, et al. Abdominal aorta: evaluation with dual-source dual-energy multidetector CT after endovascular repair of aneurysms–initial observations. Radiology 2008; 249(2):692–700.

Practical Applications of Dual-Energy Computed Tomography in the Acute Abdomen

Mohammed F. Mohammed, MBBS, CIIP[a],*,
Khaled Y. Elbanna, FRCR[b],
Abdelazim M.E. Mohammed, MBBS[a], Nicolas Murray, MD[c],
Fahad Azzumea, MBBS[a], Ghassan Almazied, MBBS[a],
Savvas Nicolaou, MD[c]

KEYWORDS

• Dual-energy CT • Abdomen • Pelvis • Trauma • Ischemia • Gangrene • Gallstone • Inflammation

KEY POINTS

- Low kiloelectron volt virtual monoenergetic image (VMI) reconstructions enable improved contrast resolution, allowing for improved assessment of organ perfusion.
- Low kiloelectron volt VMI reconstructions also allow for reduction of contrast load without sacrificing image quality.
- Dual-energy computed tomography (DECT) allows for identification of iodine, thus enabling detection of subtle hemorrhages or oral contrast extravasation.
- Virtual noncontrast images can help differentiate hematomas or calcifications from iodine without the need for further imaging.
- The ability to differentiate various materials by DECT allows for differentiation of types of renal stones and shows promise in detection of noncalcified gallstones.

INTRODUCTION

Interest in dual-energy computed tomography (DECT) has steadily increased since the introduction of the first clinical scanner in 2006. Research has particularly been focused on the role of DECT in oncological applications. Its applicability in acutely ill and injured patients was limited owing to concerns about image quality; acquisition speed; radiation dose; and, most importantly, workflow limitations requiring a large chunk of the radiologist's time. However, recent advances in DECT technologies have addressed all these issues, enabling dose-neutral (or dose-negative) scans, acquired rapidly with image quality comparable or better than conventional computed tomography (CT).[1–4] The latest software versions offered by all major CT vendors include several workflow automation options that significantly

[a] Medical Imaging Department, Abdominal Imaging Section, Ministry of the National Guard, Health Affairs, King Saud bin Abdulaziz University for Health Sciences, King Abdullah International Medical Research Center, Prince Mutib Ibn Abdullah Ibn Abdulaziz Road, Ar Rimayah, Riyadh 14611, Saudi Arabia; [b] Department of Medical Imaging, Emergency and Trauma Radiology Division, Sunnybrook Health Sciences Centre, University of Toronto, 2075 Bayview Avenue, Toronto, Ontario M4N 3M5, Canada; [c] Department of Radiology, Vancouver General Hospital, 899 West 12th Avenue, Vancouver, British Columbia V5Z1M9, Canada
* Corresponding author.
E-mail address: mohammed.f.mohammed@gmail.com

Radiol Clin N Am 56 (2018) 549–563
https://doi.org/10.1016/j.rcl.2018.03.004

reduce the time needed to produce interpretable data from dual energy datasets.

The ability of DECT to characterize materials based on their chemical composition has enabled assessment of disease processes in new ways that help improve the sensitivity and specificity of CT in the acute setting. For example, by identifying iodine, contrast can be subtracted, generating virtual noncontrast (VNC) images to detect a hematoma or confirm areas of calcification. The same technique can be used to assess organ perfusion by assessing iodine distribution within the organ of interest. Contrast extravasation is also more accurately assessed by iodine-labeling techniques. Material labeling also enables stone characterization, which has a direct impact on management. New techniques are also enabling the detection of noncalcified gallstones, adding tremendous value to CT of the abdomen and pelvis because it is usually the first study for many patients with nonspecific abdominal pain and would enable detection of gallstones in suspected cholecystitis or pancreatitis.

Virtual monoenergetic images (VMIs) allow improvement of the contrast-to-noise ratio (CNR), improving detection of subtle findings such as areas of decreased enhancement or small lacerations in trauma.

This article reviews the established applications for DECT of the abdomen and pelvis in an organ system–based approach, including how it adds value in the assessment of an acutely ill or injured patient.

GASTROINTESTINAL TRACT
Bowel Obstruction and Ischemia

The causes of small bowel ischemia include arterial occlusion (60%–70%), venous occlusion (5%–10%), strangulated bowel obstruction (10%), and low-flow states (20%). Arterial occlusion is associated with abnormally thin bowel wall with decreased enhancement but it could be thickened in the reperfusion state. On the other hand, bowel wall thickening with edema or hemorrhage occurs with venous ischemia and strangulation.[5] Other findings include mesenteric fat stranding with free fluid, pneumatosis intestinalis, and portomesenteric venous gas.[6]

The most reliable sign for diagnosis of bowel ischemia is absent or diminished bowel wall enhancement, which may be subtle on conventional CT. In a study by Potretzke and colleagues,[7] the difference in attenuation between the perfused and ischemic bowels on 120 kilovolt (peak) (kV[p]) conventional CT imaging can be doubled at 51 keV VMI. Hence, an ischemic bowel segment can be more easily distinguished from a nonischemic bowel on DECT.[8] This is important, particularly in cases of acute small bowel obstruction in which conventional CT imaging has low sensitivity to identify ischemic nonviable segments, whereas low kiloelectron volt VMI increases contrast resolution. However, because of increased noise, low kiloelectron volt VMI is best used as a complementary dataset, rather than a dataset that replaces the conventional images.[9,10] Combining them with iodine overlay (IO) images can improve sensitivity and specificity of diagnosing bowel ischemia (Figs. 1 and 2).

Inflammatory and Infectious Conditions

Inflammatory bowel diseases include ulcerative colitis, in which the inflammation is limited to the large intestine and affects only the intestinal mucosa, and Crohn disease, which can affect any part of the gastrointestinal (GI) tract, commonly the terminal ileum, and is usually transmural in nature.[11] In the acute exacerbations of active inflammatory bowel disease, abdominopelvic CT can distinguish the location and length of the inflamed segments, as well as complications such as penetrating disease and abscess.[12]

The alteration in bowel wall enhancement is accentuated at low kiloelectron volt VMI and IO images, which have a higher sensitivity in detecting subtle areas of mural hyperenhancement compared with conventional CT images.[13,14] In Crohn disease, small bowel segments with active inflammation become clearly noticeable and distinguished from the spared bowel segments by using low kiloelectron volt VMI, demonstrating mural hyperenhancement with a corresponding increase in iodine uptake on IO images (Fig. 3). Similarly, the degree of enhancement and iodine density of the inflammatory stricture are expected to be higher than the chronic fibrotic stricture.[15,16] In addition, IO images can be helpful to differentiate between enteric contrast accumulation within fistulas and hyperattenuating fluid collections.[16]

Colonic diverticulitis is demonstrated as a mild increase in enhancement of the colonic wall and adjacent fat that are reflected as increased iodine density on IO images.[13] However, this increase in iodine density was found to be significantly lower than in adenocarcinoma of the colon,[17] with a cutoff value for iodine concentration of 3 mg/mL being highly suggestive of adenocarcinoma rather than diverticulitis (Fig. 4). Primary epiploic appendagitis results from torsion of epiploic appendages, leading to ischemic infarction, and commonly appears as oval fat-density lesion abutting the colonic wall and surrounded by inflammatory changes.[18] On IO

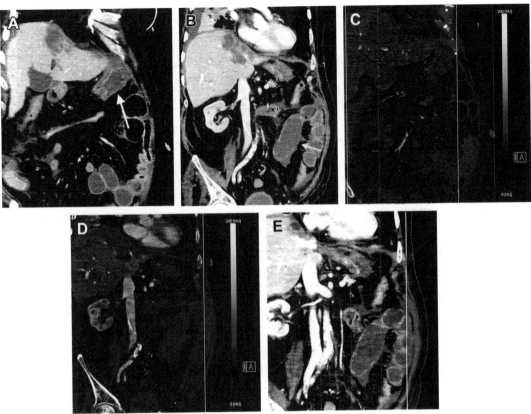

Fig. 1. An extremely ill patient with elevated lactic acid and a distended abdomen. Coronal contrast-enhanced mixed images (*A, B*) in portal venous phase shows decreased mucosal enhancement of the stomach (*white arrow*) and a faint decrease in enhancement along the antimesenteric wall of a jejunal loop (*yellow arrow*). IO images (*C, D*) confirm loss of iodine of the gastric and jejunal mucosa, confirming gastric and jejunal ischemia. A 40 keV VMI reconstruction (*E*) accentuates the lack of enhancement in the ischemic loop.

images, iodine density is diminished or absent within the infarcted appendage and its hyperdense rim, contrasting the increased iodine of the surrounding inflamed fat.[15]

Although CT has a minimal role in the diagnosis of peptic ulcer disease and upper GI tract inflammation, it is often the initial modality for workup of nonspecific abdominal pain; hence, it may be

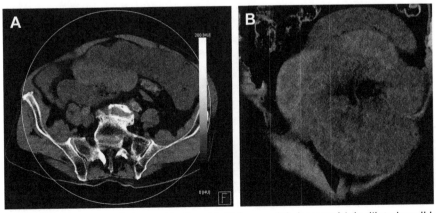

Fig. 2. A patient with vomiting and elevated lactic acid. IO images (*A*) show multiple dilated small bowel loops centrally in a sac-like configuration suggestive of a closed loop obstruction with diminished iodine uptake. The VNC images (*B*) demonstrate hyperdensity in the proximal loops, consistent with intramural hematoma. Findings were confirmed on surgery.

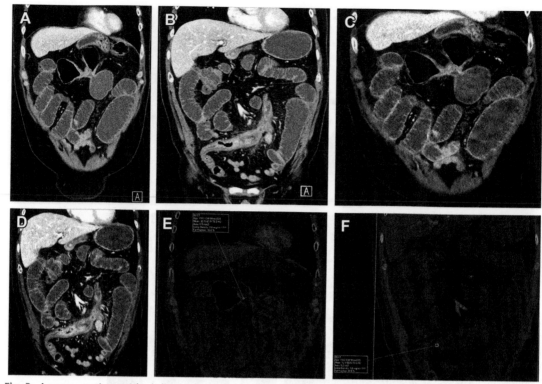

Fig. 3. A young patient with abdominal pain who is known to have Crohn disease. Coronal contrast-enhanced mixed images (*A*, *B*) in portal venous demonstrate multifocal short-segment strictures in the proximal ileal loops (*A*) and a long-segment stricture in a distal ileal loop (*B*) but show fairly similar enhancement. (*C*, *D*) 40 keV VMI reconstructions demonstrate hyperenhancement in the long-segment stricture (*D*) compared with the short-segment proximal strictures (*C*). IO images (*E*, *F*) confirm an increase in iodine density within the long-segment stricture, indicating an active inflammatory stricture.

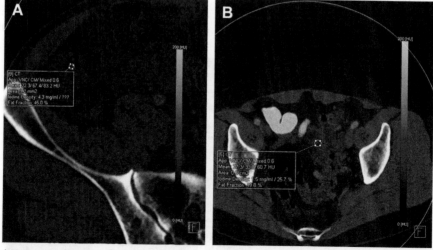

Fig. 4. Axial IO images from 2 different patients with colonic wall thickening due to adenocarcinoma (*A*) and diverticulitis (*B*), with regions of interest drawn over thickened bowel wall. The iodine density in colonic adeno-carcinoma is significantly higher (4.3 mg/mL) than in diverticulitis (1.5 mg/mL in this case). Iodine concentration of greater than 3 mg/mL is suggestive of colonic adenocarcinoma rather than diverticulitis in case of diffuse bowel wall thickening.

the first study to suggest presence of upper GI inflammation. In the presence of a distended stomach, gastric wall thickening is the most common CT finding in gastritis and the presence of mural stratification can help differentiate gastritis from malignancy.[19] On DECT IO images, absence of an underlying mass may be suggested by lack of an iodine-containing mural lesion. IO images are also helpful to accurately detect the wall hyperemia and the adjacent soft tissue inflammation in cases of duodenitis.[13] DECT may also improve detection of wall defects in cases of perforated peptic ulcer disease by demonstrating focal lack of iodine uptake on IO images or focal decreased enhancement on low kiloelectron volt VMI. IO images may also demonstrate presence of minimal oral contrast in perigastric and periduodenal fluid collections, confirming perforation with subtle contrast leak (**Fig. 5**).

Appendicitis

The diagnostic criteria of appendicitis by CT includes presence of an enlarged appendix, appendiceal wall thickening, hyperenhancement, presence of an appendicolith, and periappendiceal fat stranding.[20] IO images can demonstrate

subtle wall hyperenhancement in early appendicitis even in the absence of periappendiceal fat stranding.[13]

Based on preliminary work,[21,22] low kiloelectron volt VMI and IO images can also detect early nonperforated gangrene of the appendiceal wall, which appears as focal or diffuse loss of wall enhancement. Therefore, DECT may help identify patients who would fail conservative therapy or are at an increased risk for perforation and postoperative complications (**Fig. 6**). On the other hand, a subtle mural soft tissue nodule becomes more conspicuous on low kiloelectron volt VMI and IO images with better identification of coexisting occult appendiceal tumors. VNC imaging can differentiate a calcified fecalith from oral contrast at the base of appendix, where the former still appears as a hyperdense focus while oral contrast is subtracted.[15]

Gastrointestinal Bleeding

GI bleeding (GIB) is a common condition associated with significant morbidity and mortality. Common causes of upper GIB include mucosal erosions, peptic ulcers, tumors, and inflammatory or diverticular conditions, typically present with

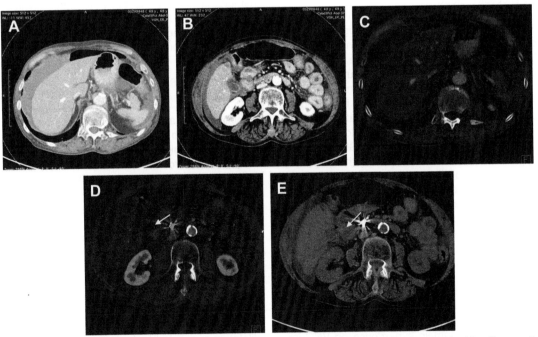

Fig. 5. Patient with sudden onset of acute abdominal pain with history of coil embolization for bleeding peptic ulcer disease. Axial contrast-enhanced mixed images (*A, B*) in the portal venous phase with oral contrast show pneumoperitoneum and a large amount of free fluid in the upper abdomen. IO images (*C, D*) demonstrate iodine in the fluid, in keeping with leaking oral contrast. A focal area of decreased iodine is noted along the lateral wall of D2 (*yellow arrows*), which is hyperdense on VNC images (*E*), in keeping with a small hematoma at the site of perforation. Findings were confirmed on surgery.

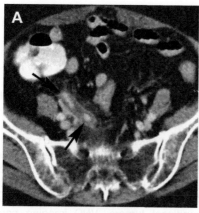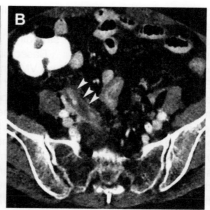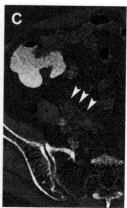

Fig. 6. Patient with 1-day history of abdominal pain. Axial contrast-enhanced mixed images (*A*) of the lower abdomen show an inflamed appendix with 2 intraluminal calcified appendicoliths (*black arrows*). No evidence of gangrene. 40 keV VMI reconstruction (*B*) demonstrates loss of mural enhancement along the anterior wall of the appendix (*arrowheads*). The IO image (*C*) demonstrates lack of iodine uptake at the gangrenous anterior wall of the appendix (*arrowheads*). Nonperforated gangrene was confirmed by histopathology.

hematemesis, melena, or coffee ground vomiting. On the other hand, angioectasia or angiodysplasia, neoplasms, inflammation, or diverticular diseases are common causes of lower GIB, frequently presenting with melena, hematochezia, or rectal bleeding. CT angiography is important for localization of active bleeding in cases of massive bleeding because the endoscopic view is limited by excessive blood.[23–25]

The contrast resolution within the vessels at the lower energy spectrum of DECT is higher than the conventional CT technique, which enables reduction of the required dose of the intravenous contrast media. Automatic or semiautomatic subtraction of vascular calcification from the enhancing vascular lumen is also improved by DECT.[26,27] VNC imaging can obviate the unenhanced phase as a part of the traditional triphasic CT protocol performed for cases of GIB, leading to dose reduction in a CT protocol with arterial and dual-energy portal venous phases by up to 30%.[28] Owing to its ability to demonstrate subtle areas of contrast extravasation and to quantify iodine in areas of suspected bleeding, IO images are more accurate than conventional CT in cases of acute GIB.[16,23] Moreover, an active bleed is demonstrated as a focus or foci of high-iodine content that are subtracted on VNC imaging, allowing for differentiation from hyperdense ingested materials, such as ingested bismuth, nonsteroidal antiinflammatory drugs, and food particles, which remain hyperdense on VNC images[13,29] (**Fig. 7**).

Spontaneous intramural small bowel hematoma can occur in patients with increased risk of bleeding, especially those who receive anticoagulant therapy. CT diagnosis of this condition can be suggested by the presence of mural hyperdensity within an area of circumferential thickening of the small bowel. Intramural hemorrhage commonly involves a short segment of small bowel and may even mimic a focal mass.[30,31] On VMI, an enhancing mass demonstrates a higher attenuation on the low-energy spectrum relative to the high-energy spectrum. Conversely, an intramural hematoma follows the opposite pattern with a higher attenuation on 140 keV VMI or more. Intramural hemorrhage remains hyperdense on VNC image reconstruction as well[15] (**Fig. 8**).

PANCREATICOBILIARY
Cholelithiasis and Cholecystitis

Cholelithiasis is a major health problem worldwide that may lead to biliary obstruction, acute cholecystitis, cholangitis, or pancreatitis. Cholelithiasis can lead to chronic proliferative cholangitis and is associated with an increased risk for cholangiocarcinoma.[32] Ultrasound is highly sensitive and specific in detecting gallstones and remains the initial imaging modality of choice in acute gallbladder disease due to accessibility, relatively short examination time, and lack of ionizing radiation. Owing to its variable composition, conventional CT has a relatively low sensitivity in detecting gallstones and large, noncalcified gallstones.[33,34]

Biliary stones indirectly manifest on CT as biliary dilatation or gallbladder hydrops. On conventional CT, calcified stones can be identified. However, cholesterol or noncalcified stones are frequently missed because their density is similar to bile at 120 kV(p) acquisitions.[35] DECT has the advantage of generating material decomposition images that

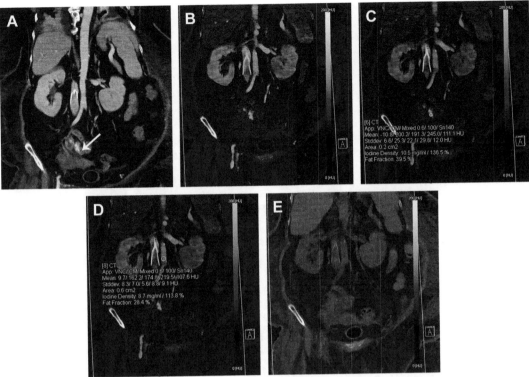

Fig. 7. Patient with bleeding per rectum and a drop in hemoglobin. Coronal contrast-enhanced mixed images (*A*) in portal venous phase show dense intraluminal material (*white arrow*). IO images (*B–D*) show accumulation of iodine with iodine density higher than the aorta confirming contrast extravasation. The extravasation is not visualized on VNC images (*E*). Patient was successfully treated by embolization.

can be used to differentiate similarly attenuating materials of differing chemical compositions from each other. Additionally, low kiloelectron volt or high kiloelectron volt VMI reconstructions can accentuate the subtle attenuation differences between bile and noncalcified gallstones. A 40 keV VMI is superior to a conventional CT image in gallstones visualization, especially noncalcified stones. Similar performance has been demonstrated on calcium-based material decomposition images. These techniques were also superior to 140 keV VMI and lipid-based material decomposition images.[35,36]

Kim and colleagues[32] investigated the added value of VNC images for detection of biliary stones. VNC imaging is an acceptable substitute for true noncontrast imaging. VNC imaging allows the detection of biliary stones with moderate accuracy, irrespective of the dual-energy contrast-enhanced phase, with limited diagnostic value for stones less than 1.7 mm or stones of 78 HU or lower.

Li and colleagues[37] emphasized the value of rapid switching DECT (rsDECT) in detection of noncalcified stones with 100% accuracy with the utility of calcium-based and lipid-based material decomposition, optimal CNR VMI, and spectral curve images. On rsDECT, the mean attenuation difference between noncalcified stones and adjacent bile is significantly higher on optimal VMI (47.30 HU) than on conventional CT images (6.87 HU). Material decomposition imaging highlights the differences in calcium and fat concentrations between the bile and noncalcified stone. As a result, a noncalcified stone with its lower calcium content appears as a dark spot on calcium-based images, in contrast to a bright spot identified on a fat-based image due to its high lipid content. Similar results have been reported in a recent study by Yang and colleagues,[36] who concluded that a lipid concentration of 182.59 mg/mL could be used as a cutoff level to discriminate noncalcified gallstones from bile with 95.5% sensitivity, 100% specificity, and 99% accuracy. The attenuation of cholesterol stone was lowest at 40 keV and peaked at 140 keV VMI, in contradistinction to the spectral behavior of bile, allowing for improved detection of the stone. This peculiar spectral behavior of noncalcified gallstones was also identified on dual source DECT (dsDECT), in which 40 keV VMI showed the highest attenuation difference between the noncalcified stones and

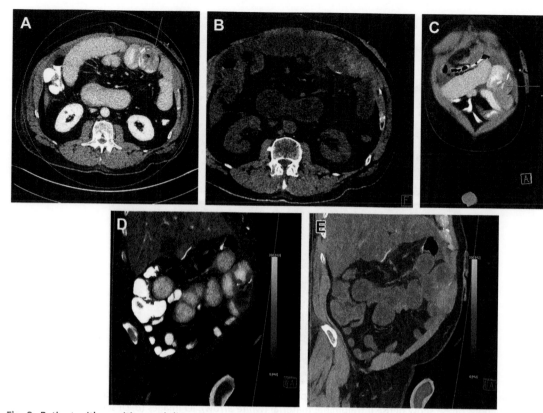

Fig. 8. Patient with vomiting and distention post-Roux-en-Y. Axial contrast-enhanced mixed image (*A*) in portal venous phase demonstrates a hypodense filling defect at the jejunojejunal anastomosis (*grey arrow*) with biliary loop dilatation (afferent loop syndrome). VNC image (*B*) reveals that the filling defect is hyperdense, in keeping with a hematoma. Coronal mixed (*C*) and IO (*D*) images demonstrate an iodine-containing linear hyperdensity at the anastomosis (*white arrow, C*), which disappears on VNC images (*E*), in keeping with active extravasation at the anastomosis. Findings were confirmed at surgery.

bile of more than 20 HU in 100% of stones and 44 HU in 75%. On the contrary, 78% of noncalcified gallstones were unidentifiable on 70 keV VMI, which simulates conventional 120 kV(p) imaging.[38] Preliminary work by O'Connell and colleagues using the dsDECT platform has shown promise in detecting gallstones using a lipid-based material decomposition technique.[39]

Ultrasound has a limited diagnostic value in the evaluation of complicated acute cholecystitis that may require CT or MR imaging for accurate localization and surgical planning. On CT, uncomplicated acute cholecystitis manifests as an overdistended gallbladder with wall thickening, pericholecystic fat stranding, pericholecystic fluid, and hyperemia of the adjacent liver parenchyma.[33,34] Gangrenous cholecystitis may complicate acute calculous cholecystitis and eventually lead to gallbladder perforation. CT findings of markedly distended gallbladder and decreased wall enhancement have an approximately 92% specificity and an approximately 89% accuracy to predict gangrenous cholecystitis.[40]

DECT with IO images of iodine material density displays can clearly reflect the subtle differences in enhancement.[41] In the authors' experience, this can help demonstrate subtle hyperenhancement of the gallbladder wall and adjacent hepatic hyperemia in cases of acute cholecystitis and aid detection of mural loss of enhancement in gangrenous cholecystitis (**Fig. 9**).

Gallstone ileus is a rare complication of cholecystitis that presents as intestinal obstruction due to an impacted ectopic gallstone, usually in the distal ileum.[33,34] DECT, with its ability to visualize the noncalcified stone, can help localize an impacted stone that may be unidentified on conventional CT.[35]

Pancreas

In cases of pancreatitis, DECT is mainly required to assess for complications, including pancreatic necrosis, pancreatic or peripancreatic collections, and vascular complications. CT images reconstructed at low kiloelectron volt values using VMI can help detect pancreatic necrosis with improved

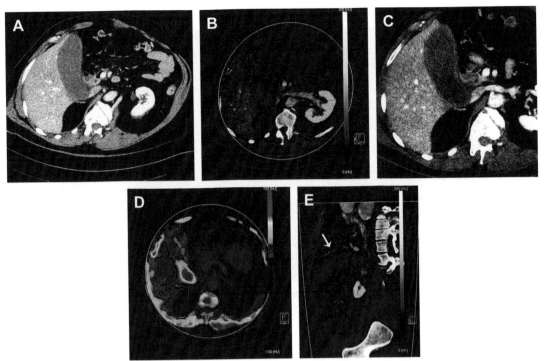

Fig. 9. Patient with diffuse abdominal pain. Axial contrast-enhanced mixed images (*A*) in portal venous phase shows distended gallbladder with slightly thickened wall. IO images (*B*) demonstrate lack of iodine uptake along the medial wall of the neck, which is better demonstrated on 40 keV VMI reconstructions (*C*), suggestive of focal gangrene or necrosis. Lipid-based material decomposition image (*D*) demonstrates cholesterol containing gallstone (*red*) with surrounding bile (*purple-green*). Sagittal IO images (*E*) show pericholecystic hyperemia within the surrounding hepatic parenchyma (*white arrow*) in the form of increased iodine density. Findings were confirmed intraoperatively.

CNR and better subjective assessment compared with 120 kV imaging owing to its advantage of accentuating subtle differences in enhancement, and aids in the diagnosis of venous thrombosis and arterial pseudoaneurysms.[42,43] Furthermore, DECT can provide further discrimination of decreased perfusion from necrosis due to accurate delineation of iodine distribution in the inflamed pancreatic tissue.[41] VNC imaging can also be used to detect pancreatic calcifications without obtaining a true unenhanced CT, reducing radiation and study time.[16]

Distinguishing pancreatic adenocarcinoma from chronic mass-forming pancreatitis (CMFP) is challenging even on histopathology, and the incidence of focal pancreatitis can be up to 13% in patients undergoing surgery for clinically suspected cancer.[44] On DECT, iodine density and K slope have been reported to be higher in CMFP than in pancreatic adenocarcinoma on both arterial and portal venous phases. The reported mean normalized iodine concentration and mean spectral curve slope of the CMFP and adenocarcinoma is 0.53 versus 0.28, and 3.7 versus 2.16 on the portal venous phase, respectively. The iodine concentration of

the lesion is normalized to the iodine concentration of the aorta and K slope on VMI CT values is defined as CT (90 keV) – CT (40 keV)/50. The difference of iodine density in both entities could be due to relatively abundant neovascularization in fresh CMFP or dense fibrotic tissue in advanced CMFP leading to more iodine accumulation in the lesion.[43,45]

GENITOURINARY
Nephrolithiasis

The chemical composition of the urinary calculi affects patient management and can also predict the likelihood of stone recurrence. single energy CT (SECT) can detect and localize symptomatic urinary calculi. However, it has moderate accuracy in differentiating stone composition. DECT as a noninvasive imaging tool can help characterize the chemical composition of urinary stones.[46–48] This advantage of DECT is provided without increasing the radiation dose or affecting image quality.[49]

Using material decomposition algorithms, DECT is able to characterize urinary calculi by 2 different methods. On rsDECT, urate calculi are visualized only on material-specific water images, whereas

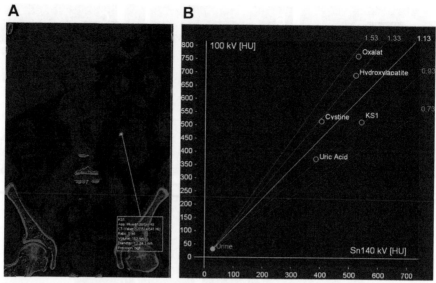

Fig. 10. Patient with recurrent renal stones. Coronal dual energy CT material decomposition image (*A*) demonstrating a uric acid stone. Note that the stone lies on the uric acid identity line (*B*). Calcium-containing stones would be colored blue.

nonurate stones are visualized on both material-specific iodine and water images.[50] On dsDECT and dual-layer detector DECT, differentiation of stones is based on the calculation of the DECT number ratio, defined as a ratio of the CT number of a given material at low-to-high energy spectra.[51] Automated material decomposition software for DECT can separate the main chemical constituents of renal calculi, which include water (urine), calcium, and uric acid. The spectral behavior of each calculus is demonstrated as a specific slope and assigned a certain color on a color-coded map; for example, purple-blue for nonurate calcium-containing calculi and red for urate-based calculi[48,52] (**Fig. 10**).

DECT has better accuracy in distinguishing uric acid calculi from nonuric acid calculi (90%–100%).[51] In modern dsDECT systems, applying additional tin (Sn) filtration to the high-energy spectrum (Sn140 kV or Sn150 kV) increases the separation of the dual-energy spectra and allows further subcategorization of nonuric acid stones, such as calcium oxalate (monohydrate or dihydrate), cystine, struvite, and hydroxyapatite stones.[16,46] Combining tin filtration and higher energies for the low-energy tube (90 or 100 kV as opposed to 80 kV) enables accurate stone characterization, even for smaller stones, without sacrificing image quality.[48,53]

Adrenal Lesions

There are limited acute conditions that affect the adrenal glands. Adrenal hemorrhage is uncommon condition; however, traumatic is more common than nontraumatic hemorrhage, which can be due

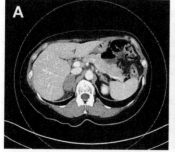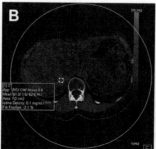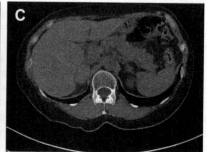

Fig. 11. Patient post-MVC. Axial contrast-enhanced mixed images (*A*) in portal venous phase show a nonspecific right adrenal lesion. IO images (*B*) demonstrate lack of iodine uptake in the lesion. The lesion is hyperdense on VNC images (*C*), confirming an adrenal hematoma without active bleeding.

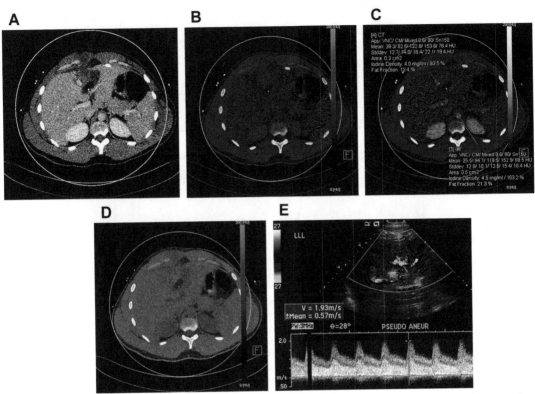

Fig. 12. Patient after a motor vehicle collision. Axial contrast-enhanced mixed images (A) in portal venous phase demonstrate a geographic low-attenuation area at segment IV of the liver, in keeping with a laceration, and an eccentric high-attenuation focus. Color-coded IO image (B) shows increased iodine density in the eccentric high-attenuation focus but does not exceed that of the aorta (C), with no increase in iodine density in the laceration, confirming a pseudoaneurysm. The pseudoaneurysm is not appreciated on VNC images (D), confirming iodine content. Doppler ultrasound (E) confirms presence of a pseudoaneurysm, which was successfully treated by coil embolization.

to stress, intratumoral hemorrhage, and bleeding disorders. Unenhanced CT shows a hyperdense mass with surrounding fat stranding.[54] Adrenal hemorrhage in the acute setting can be easily and accurately diagnosable by DECT. VNC images reveal hyperdensity in the adrenal lesion, whereas IO images would show no contrast uptake in the lesion, confirming an adrenal hematoma without the need for further workup[52] (Fig. 11).

TRAUMA

CT is the main diagnostic study in assessment of the hemodynamically stable patient with trauma to the abdomen or pelvis.[55] DECT adds value in trauma patients in several ways. The authors' protocol for scanning abdominal trauma consists of an ultrahigh pitch angiographic arterial acquisition followed by a dual-energy portal venous phase acquisition. Delayed images are acquired selectively at the discretion of the attending radiologist at the time of the scan.

In cases with pelvic fractures, differentiating contrast extravasation from osseous fragments can be challenging; however, VNC imaging with its ability to subtract and eliminate iodinated contrast material adds diagnostic value in such cases, in which osseous fragments remain hyperdense on VNC imaging. Active arterial bleeding can be readily identified on color-coded IO images as areas of iodine density higher than that of the abdominal aorta during the portal venous phase. Thus, subtle foci of active bleeding can be easily detected on IO images.[15,56] On the other hand, a traumatic pseudoaneurysm is expected to follow the enhancement pattern of the abdominal aorta.[57] Delayed phase DECT with IO images improves subjective detection of slow flow venous bleeding that is not obvious on arterial and portal venous phases, which is demonstrated as insidiously increased iodine density on the delayed images.[15,56] Low kiloelectron volt VMI reconstructions are used to improve detection of subtle lacerations by improving CNR (Figs. 12–14).

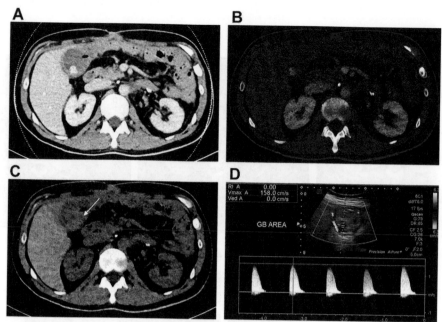

Fig. 13. Young male patient with bloody discharge through a suspected enterocutaneous fistula with a history of gunshot wound. Portal venous phase mixed images (*A*) demonstrate a dependent focus of hyperdensity within the gallbladder, as well as air along the nondependent portion, related to a traumatic cholecystoenteric fistula. The hyperdensity consists of iodine similar to that of the blood-pool as demonstrated on IO images (*B*) and is not appreciated on VNC images; however, a surrounding hematoma is noted within the gallbladder lumen (*white arrow*) (*C*), in keeping with a pseudoaneurysm. Doppler ultrasound (*D*) confirmed presence of a traumatic cystic artery pseudoaneurysm and was subsequently treated by coil embolization.

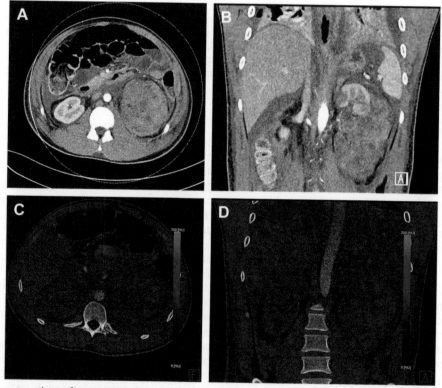

Fig. 14. Young patient after trauma while mountain biking. Contrast-enhanced mixed images (*A*, *B*) in arterial phase show a shattered left kidney with residual enhancement involving the renal cortex. A large perinephric hematoma is present. IO images (*C*, *D*) confirm renal perfusion with no areas of iodine uptake within the hematoma to suggest active extravasation. The findings are in keeping with a grade IV injury.

VMI and IO images can be used to assess bowel perfusion as previously described. This improves detection of bowel injury, which may demonstrate hypoperfusion, diminished enhancement, or mural hyperdensity due to an intramural hematoma, which can be readily identified on DECT, especially in the absence of other signs, such as pneumoperitoneum or enteric contrast leak.[8,15,58,59]

REFERENCES

1. Foley WD, Shuman WP, Siegel MJ, et al. White paper of the Society of Computed Body Tomography and Magnetic Resonance on dual-energy CT, part 2: radiation dose and iodine sensitivity. J Comput Assist Tomogr 2016;40(6):846–50.

2. Uhrig M, Simons D, Kachelrieß M, et al. Advanced abdominal imaging with dual energy CT is feasible without increasing radiation dose. Cancer Imaging 2016;16(1):15.

3. Purysko AS, Primak AN, Baker ME, et al. Comparison of radiation dose and image quality from single-energy and dual-energy CT examinations in the same patients screened for hepatocellular carcinoma. Clin Radiol 2014;69(12):e538–44.

4. Shuman WP, Green DE, Busey JM, et al. Dual-energy liver CT: effect of monochromatic imaging on lesion detection, conspicuity, and contrast-to-noise ratio of hypervascular lesions on late arterial phase. Am J Roentgenol 2014;203(3):601–6.

5. Furukawa A, Kanasaki S, Kono N, et al. CT diagnosis of acute mesenteric ischemia from various causes. Am J Roentgenol 2009;192(2):408–16.

6. Dhatt HS, Behr SC, Miracle A, et al. Radiological evaluation of bowel ischemia. Radiol Clin North Am 2015;53(6):1241–54.

7. Potretzke TA, Brace CL, Lubner MG, et al. Early small-bowel ischemia: dual-energy ct improves conspicuity compared with conventional CT in a swine model. Radiology 2015;275(1):119–26.

8. Wallace AB, Raptis CA, Mellnick VM. Imaging of bowel ischemia. Curr Radiol Rep 2016;4(6):29.

9. Lourenco P, Rawski R, McLaughlin PD, et al. Dual-energy CT and virtual monoenergetic reconstructions: utility of novel and basic algorithms in assessment of intestinal wall enhancement and applications for acute intestinal ischemia. Paper presented at: Radiological Society of North America 2015, 101st Scientific Assembly and Annual Meeting. Chicago (IL), November 29–December 4, 2015. [Abstract: RC509-06]. n.d.

10. Darras KE, McLaughlin PD, Kang H, et al. Virtual monoenergetic reconstruction of contrast-enhanced dual energy CT at 70keV maximizes mural enhancement in acute small bowel obstruction. Eur J Radiol 2016;85(5):950–6.

11. Kilcoyne A, Kaplan JL, Gee MS. Inflammatory bowel disease imaging: current practice and future directions. World J Gastroenterol 2016;22(3):917.

12. Elsayes KM, Al-Hawary MM, Jagdish J, et al. CT enterography: principles, trends, and interpretation of findings. Radiographics 2010;30(7):1955–70.

13. Fulwadhva UP, Wortman JR, Sodickson AD. Use of dual-energy CT and iodine maps in evaluation of bowel disease. Radiographics 2016;36(2):393–406.

14. Apfaltrer P, Meyer M, Meier C, et al. Contrast-enhanced dual-energy CT of gastrointestinal stromal tumors: is iodine-related attenuation a potential indicator of tumor response? Invest Radiol 2012;47(1): 65–70.

15. Ali IT, Thomas C, Elbanna KY, et al. Gastrointestinal imaging: emerging role of dual-energy computed tomography. Curr Radiol Rep 2017;5(8):31.

16. Patino M, Prochowski A, Agrawal MD, et al. Material separation using dual-energy CT: current and emerging applications. Radiographics 2016;36(4): 1087–105.

17. Darras K, Clark SJ, Kang H, et al. Colonic wall thickening: can iodine quantification using dual source dual energy CT differentiate diverticulitis from adenocarcinoma? Paper presented at: Radiological Society of North America 2016, 102nd Scientific Assembly and Annual Meeting. Chicago (IL), November 27–December 2, 2016. [Abstract: SSE06-04].

18. Singh AK, Gervais DA, Hahn PF, et al. Acute epiploic appendagitis and its mimics. Radiographics 2005; 25(6):1521–34.

19. Guniganti P, Bradenham CH, Raptis C, et al. CT of gastric emergencies. Radiographics 2015;35(7): 1909–21.

20. Pinto Leite N, Pereira JM, Cunha R, et al. CT evaluation of appendicitis and its complications: imaging techniques and key diagnostic findings. Am J Roentgenol 2005;185(2):406–17.

21. Mohammed MF, Elbanna KY, Chahal TS, et al. Imaging of gangrenous appendicitis: do dual energy iodine overlay images add clinical value?. Paper presented at: Radiological Society of North America 2017, 103rd Scientific Assembly and Annual Meeting. Chicago (IL), November 26–December 1, 2017. [Abstract: SSQ07-08].

22. Mohammed MF, Elbanna KY, Chahal TS, et al. Imaging of gangrenous appendicitis: do dual energy virtual monoenergetic images add clinical value?. Paper presented at: Radiological Society of North America 2017, 103rd Scientific Assembly and Annual Meeting. Chicago (IL). November 26–December 1, 2017. [Abstract: RC508-04]. n.d.

23. Sun H, Hou X-Y, Xue H-D, et al. Dual-source dual-energy CT angiography with virtual non-enhanced images and iodine map for active gastrointestinal bleeding: image quality, radiation dose and

diagnostic performance. Eur J Radiol 2015;84(5): 884–91.

24. Geffroy Y, Rodallec MH, Boulay-Coletta I, et al. Multidetector CT angiography in acute gastrointestinal bleeding: why, when, and how. Radiographics 2011;31(3):E35–46.

25. Graça BM, Freire PA, Brito JB, et al. Gastroenterologic and radiologic approach to obscure gastrointestinal bleeding: how, why, and when? Radiographics 2010;30(1):235–52.

26. Yeh BM, Shepherd JA, Wang ZJ, et al. Dual-energy and low-kVp CT in the abdomen. Am J Roentgenol 2009;193(1):47–54.

27. Coursey CA, Nelson RC, Boll DT, et al. Dual-energy multidetector CT: how does it work, what can it tell us, and when can we use it in abdominopelvic imaging? Radiographics 2010;30(4):1037–55.

28. Artigas JM, Martí M, Soto JA, et al. Multidetector CT angiography for acute gastrointestinal bleeding: technique and findings. Radiographics 2013;33(5): 1453–70.

29. De Cecco CN, Boll DT, Bolus DN, et al. White paper of the society of computed body tomography and magnetic resonance on dual-energy CT, part 4: abdominal and pelvic applications. J Comput Assist Tomogr 2017;41(1):8–14.

30. Abbas MA, Collins JM, Olden KW. Spontaneous intramural small-bowel hematoma: imaging findings and outcome. Am J Roentgenol 2002;179(6): 1389–94.

31. Macari M, Chandarana H, Balthazar E, et al. Intestinal ischemia versus intramural hemorrhage: CT evaluation. Am J Roentgenol 2003;180(1):177–84.

32. Kim JE, Lee JM, Baek JH, et al. Initial assessment of dual-energy CT in patients with gallstones or bile duct stones: can virtual nonenhanced images replace true nonenhanced images? Am J Roentgenol 2012;198(4):817–24.

33. Chawla A, Bosco JI, Lim TC, et al. Imaging of acute cholecystitis and cholecystitis-associated complications in the emergency setting. Singapore Med J 2015;56(8):438.

34. Shakespear JS, Shaaban AM, Rezvani M. CT findings of acute cholecystitis and its complications. Am J Roentgenol 2010;194(6):1523–9.

35. Chen A-L, Liu A-L, Wang S, et al. Detection of gallbladder stones by dual-energy spectral computed tomography imaging. World J Gastroenterol 2015; 21(34):9993.

36. Yang C-B, Zhang S, Jia Y-J, et al. Clinical application of dual-energy spectral computed tomography in detecting cholesterol gallstones from surrounding bile. Acad Radiol 2017;24(4):478–82.

37. Li H, He D, Lao Q, et al. Clinical value of spectral CT in diagnosis of negative gallstones and common bile duct stones. Abdom Imaging 2015; 40(6):1587–94.

38. Uyeda JW, Richardson IJ, Sodickson AD. Making the invisible visible: improving conspicuity of noncalcified gallstones using dual-energy CT. Abdom Radiol (NY) 2017;42(12):2933–9.

39. O'Connell T, McLaughlin PD, Khosa F, et al. Seeing is believing: visualization of radiolucent gallstones on dual-energy CT. Paper presented at: Radiological Society of North America 2016, 102nd Scientific Assembly and Annual Meeting. Chicago (IL), November 27–December 2, 2016. [Abstract: RC208-06].

40. Chang W-C, Sun Y, Wu E-H, et al. CT findings for detecting the presence of gangrenous ischemia in cholecystitis. Am J Roentgenol 2016;207(2):302–9.

41. Silva AC, Morse BG, Hara AK, et al. Dual-energy (spectral) CT: applications in abdominal imaging. Radiographics 2011;31(4):1031–46.

42. Yuan Y, Huang ZX, Li ZL, et al. Dual-source dual-energy computed tomography imaging of acute necrotizing pancreatitis–preliminary study. Sichuan Da Xue Xue Bao Yi Xue Ban 2011;42(5):691–4.

43. George E, Wortman JR, Fulwadhva UP, et al. Dual energy CT applications in pancreatic pathologies. Br J Radiol 2017;90(1080):20170411.

44. Kennedy T, Preczewski L, Stocker SJ, et al. Incidence of benign inflammatory disease in patients undergoing whipple procedure for clinically suspected carcinoma: a single-institution experience. Am J Surg 2006;191(3):437–41.

45. Yin Q, Zou X, Zai X, et al. Pancreatic ductal adenocarcinoma and chronic mass-forming pancreatitis: differentiation with dual-energy MDCT in spectral imaging mode. Eur J Radiol 2015;84(12):2470–6.

46. Wang X-G, Fan B, Wang W, et al. The value of performing dual-source dual-energy computed tomography in analysis strategy for urinary mixed stone. Int J Clin Exp Pathol 2017;10(2):1519–28.

47. Thomas C, Heuschmid M, Schilling D, et al. Urinary calculi composed of uric acid, cystine, and mineral salts: differentiation with dual-energy CT at a radiation dose comparable to that of intravenous pyelography. Radiology 2010;257(2):402–9.

48. Mileto A, Marin D. Dual-energy computed tomography in genitourinary imaging. Radiol Clin North Am 2017;55(2):373–91.

49. Jepperson MA, Cernigliaro JG, Ibrahim E-SH, et al. In vivo comparison of radiation exposure of dual-energy CT versus low-dose CT versus standard CT for imaging urinary calculi. J Endourol 2015;29(2): 141–6.

50. Kulkarni NM, Eisner BH, Pinho DF, et al. Determination of renal stone composition in phantom and patients using single-source dual-energy computed tomography. J Comput Assist Tomogr 2013;37(1): 37–45.

51. Kaza RK, Ananthakrishnan L, Kambadakone A, et al. Update of dual-energy CT applications in the

genitourinary tract. Am J Roentgenol 2017;208(6): 1185–92.

52. McCollough CH, Leng S, Yu L, et al. Dual- and multi-energy CT: principles, technical approaches, and clinical applications. Radiology 2015;276(3):637–53.

53. Duan X, Li Z, Yu L, et al. Characterization of urinary stone composition by use of third-generation dual-source dual-energy CT with increased spectral separation. Am J Roentgenol 2015;205(6):1203–7.

54. Hammond NA, Lostumbo A, Adam SZ, et al. Imaging of adrenal and renal hemorrhage. Abdom Imaging 2015;40(7):2747–60.

55. Shanmuganathan K, Mirvis SE, Chiu WC, et al. Penetrating torso trauma: triple-contrast helical CT in peritoneal violation and organ injury—a prospective study in 200 patients. Radiology 2004; 231(3):775–84.

56. Uyeda JW, Patino M, Sahani DV. Dual-energy CT in the acute abdomen. Curr Radiol Rep 2015; 3(6):20.

57. Stuhlfaut JW, Anderson SW, Soto JA. Blunt abdominal trauma: current imaging techniques and CT findings in patients with solid organ, bowel, and mesenteric injury. Semin Ultrasound CT MR 2007; 28:115–29. Elsevier.

58. Brofman N, Atri M, Hanson JM, et al. Evaluation of bowel and mesenteric blunt trauma with multidetector CT. Radiographics 2006;26(4):1119–31.

59. Soto JA, Anderson SW. Multidetector CT of blunt abdominal trauma. Radiology 2012;265(3):678–93.

The Role of Dual-Energy Computed Tomography in Assessment of Abdominal Oncology and Beyond

Desiree E. Morgan, MD

KEYWORDS

- Dual energy CT • Oncologic imaging • Low keV images • Iodine concentration • Cancer

KEY POINTS

- Dual energy computed tomography 50 keV simulated monoenergetic images and iodine material density images should be routinely viewed to improve detection and characterization of focal pancreatic lesions.
- Dual energy computed tomography 50 keV simulated monoenergetic images and iodine material density images are used to improve detection of focal hepatic lesions.
- Identification of iodine in renal lesions is equally sensitive and more specific than standard Hounsfield unit enhancement to identify renal neoplasms.
- For incidentally discovered adrenal masses, benign lesions can be confirmed on a single postcontrast dual energy computed tomography image and obviate the need for further imaging.

INTRODUCTION

Dual energy computed tomography (DECT) applications have been investigated in various tumors from head to toe. Many of the earliest clinical experiences with DECT involved the study of patients with cancer, and now with more than 10 years of experience, this modality is well-established, particularly for soft tissue tumors in the abdomen. It is important at the outset of this article to note that, just as for all patients but particularly pertinent for the cancer population, which undergoes repeated imaging surveillances, exposure to ionizing radiation should be minimized and this is achievable in the practice of DECT.[1] It has been shown that abdominal DECT is feasible without increasing radiation dose or sacrificing image quality,[2] and many have reported this technology to produce dose neutral or dose negative exposure profiles compared with conventional single energy CT.[3,4]

DECT allows for qualitative and quantitative analysis of tissue composition beyond the standard anatomic evaluation available with conventional single energy CT. Especially advantageous in patients with neoplasms is the ability of the radiologist to interrogate iodine concentration captured in DECT image data, or to increase the contribution of iodine signal to the image by viewing of lower energy simulated monoenergetic reconstructed images, which increase lesion conspicuity.[1,5] In addition to improving detection and characterization of suspected tumors, DECT may provide early evaluation of therapeutic response that is more accurate than standard anatomic size-based treatment monitoring.[6] One way this may be achieved is by using a quantitative iodine concentration rather than standard perfusion CT biomarkers,[7–9] a strategy that also results in a large reduction in radiation exposure to patients.

Department of Radiology University of Alabama at Birmingham, 619 19th Street South, JTN 456, Birmingham, AL 35249-6830, USA
E-mail address: dmorgan@uabmc.edu

Radiol Clin N Am 56 (2018) 565–585
https://doi.org/10.1016/j.rcl.2018.03.005

Another benefit of DECT involves the potential reduction in the amount of intravenous iodinated contrast administered to patients.[1] This practice is coupled with the use of viewing lower energy simulated monoenergetic reconstructed images to preserve image contrast, contrast-to-noise ratios (CNR) and signal-to-noise ratios. In 1 study, a 50% decrease in intravenous iodine concentration administered during DECT did not adversely affect the CNR in an animal model of hypervascular liver lesions when monoenergetic images ranging from 40 to 140 KV were used.[10] Phantom studies have shown that viewing of low-energy simulated monoenergetic images is helpful and can be performed with preservation of image quality, even in large patients[11] (**Fig. 1**), although many centers do limit the size of patients undergoing DECT.

Finally, the use of spectral imaging information combined with color-coded maps or filters is beneficial for the detection and characterization of neoplastic lesions,[12] and the practitioner using DECT will have to learn to optimize these new postprocessing methods in addition to becoming familiar with the nomenclature of a new CT practice environment.[13] This article summarizes the advantageous aspects of DECT as well as challenges to successful implementation in clinical practice, using an organ-based approach to various neoplasms and focusing on the abdomen while applicable throughout the body.

ABDOMINAL NEOPLASMS
Pancreas

One of the earliest applications of DECT in oncology was for evaluation of pancreatic ductal adenocarcinoma. Macari and colleagues[14] first showed that viewing 80 kVp images obtained with a first-generation dual source DECT produced better conspicuity of tumors compared with blended 120 kVp images when patients with pancreatic cancer were scanned in portal venous phase. Patel and colleagues[15] first reported the benefits of doubling tumor to nontumoral Hounsfield units differences when viewing simulated monoenergetic images at 52 keV compared with the "pictorial archive and communication system (PACS) equivalent" 70 keV images using a rapid kV switching DECT scanner when patients with pancreatic cancer were scanned in the pancreatic parenchymal phase. This same group later showed with a multireader study that agreement for objective image quality measurements was highest at 52 keV, subjective reader confidence and lesion conspicuity were best using iodine

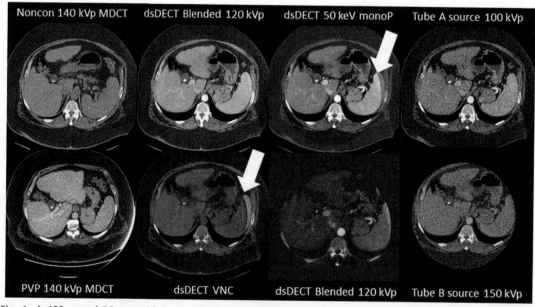

Fig. 1. A 409-pound 56-year-old man undergoing multiphasic abdominal dual energy computed tomography (DECT) for hepatocellular carcinoma surveillance. Dual source DECT image set obtained in late hepatic arterial phase demonstrates reasonable image quality on blended, low keV, and virtual noncontrast images, including visualization of the small gallstone on all images. No suspicious hepatic mass was seen. Note that the smaller of the 2 tubes (tube B, *lower right*) does not cover the full anatomic area of this large patient, resulting in the demarcation of dual from single energy image signal (*arrow*); however, the critical structures are included in the 35-cm field of view.

material density (MD) images, and overall subjective image quality was rated the highest at 70 keV.[16] The preference for lower energy simulated monoenergetic image viewing and use of iodine MD images when evaluating patients with pancreatic lesions on all major dual energy systems used in clinical practice today has now been shown by many groups[17–20] and is predominantly used for lesion detection. Becoming acquainted with the optimal CT windows and levels to view these new types of images is a challenge and there are differences among the vendors, whether the images are viewed on PACS or on the independent work stations/client servers of these systems (Fig. 2). The benefits of DECT for the detection of primary pancreatic ductal adenocarcinomas have been described whether DECT is applied during pancreatic parenchymal or portal venous phases.[21,22] The application of DECT for improved TNM staging or prediction of

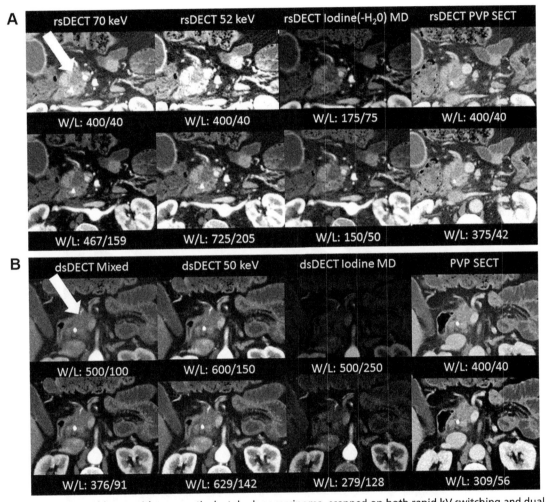

Fig. 2. A 57-year-old man with pancreatic ductal adenocarcinoma, scanned on both rapid kV switching and dual source dual energy computed tomography (DECT) scanners during pancreatic parenchymal phase. (A) Rapid kV switching DECT image set depicting a single 2.5-mm axial image with different reconstructions used for standard clinical interpretation at the author's institution. The tumor (arrow) to nontumor pancreas conspicuity is increased on the 52 keV and iodine images, which on the upper row are presented at standard window and level, and on the lower row are presented at more optimal window and level settings. (B) Dual source DECT image set through the same level of the mass (arrow) approximately 8 weeks after neoadjuvant therapy. Compare the 50-keV "monoenergetic plus" and iodine series to the blended image. Although some practices choose to view only the blended image for diagnostic interpretation, the reconstructions demonstrated in this example are all used for clinical interpretation routinely at the author's institution. Note again the difference between standard window and level on the upper row and more optimal window and level selected by the interpreter on the lower row.

an R0 resection has been less well-studied and is an area in need of more investigation, particularly the potential improvement in detection of hypovascular liver metastases in these patients. The evaluation of response to therapy in patients with pancreatic cancer is important, especially after neoadjuvant therapy or when novel treatments such as irreversible electrophoresis are used. Lower energy simulated monoenergetic images may aid in texture analysis during therapy. Although some of these topics have been described or reported in meetings,[23] there are no published papers to date.

Just as the conspicuity of hypovascular pancreatic ductal adenocarcinoma is improved when viewing lower energy or iodine MD images, sensitivity for the detection of hypervascular pancreatic neoplasms such as neuroendocrine neoplasms is improved when using lower keV and iodine MD images[24,25] (Fig. 3). Identification of multiple primary pancreatic neuroendocrine lesions as well as hypervascular liver metastases is improved with the same utilization of lower keV and iodine MD images, and color filters to enhance visualization of these lesions may be applied to either iodine or lower keV images (Fig. 4). The latter is critical,

because clinical practice now includes metastectomies for up to 5 lesions in addition to resection of the primary pancreatic endocrine tumor in efforts to control symptoms. In patients with cystic pancreatic neoplasms, the visualization of septations and nodules is improved with DECT (Fig. 5). Finally, use of individual patient CNR optimized energy levels and normalized iodine content improved sensitivity and specificity for differentiating chronic mass forming pancreatitis from pancreatic ductal adenocarcinoma.[26]

Key points: pancreas neoplasms

DECT 50 keV simulated monoenergetic images and iodine MD images are complementary to PACS equivalent images, whether 70 to 77 keV images or linear blended images, and these images should be routinely viewed clinically to improve detection of focal pancreatic lesions.

Liver

Early investigations of DECT applications of the liver focused on the detection of hypervascular hepatic lesions. Several groups identified that there were improved lesion CNRs and comparable detection sensitivities using lower energies,[27–29]

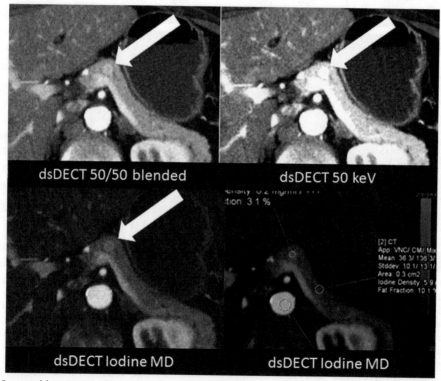

Fig. 3. A 49-year-old woman with very small pancreatic endocrine neoplasm. Dual source dual energy computed tomography image set obtained in pancreatic parenchymal phase demonstrates visualization of the tiny mass (*arrow*) in the anterior aspect of the pancreatic neck. The colorized iodine image allows for quantitative assessment of lesion iodine by placement of a region of interest.

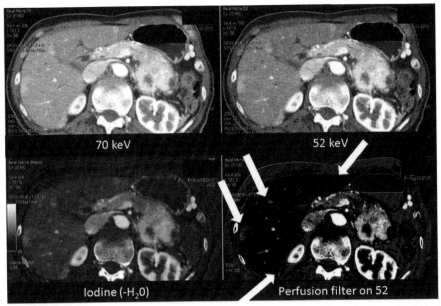

Fig. 4. A 72-year-old woman with a pancreatic endocrine neoplasm metastatic to the liver. Rapid keV switching dual energy computed tomography image set obtained in pancreatic parenchymal phase demonstrates the hyperenhancing mass expanding the pancreatic body and tail, as well as 4 hypervascular metastases (*arrows*) in the hepatic periphery. Note that these are much better depicted on all 3 dual energy images compared with the un-enhanced and portal venous phase single energy multidetector computed tomography images in the first column.

which then translated to improved lesion detection sensitivity and image quality,[30] and finally established that, as in the pancreas, viewing lower keV simulated monoenergetic images helps to identify the greatest number of lesions[4] (**Fig. 6**). Also similar to the pancreas, early trials evaluated mixed tube potential image datasets using the dual source dual energy system compared with 80 or 140 kVp source images,[31] but later efforts were engaged in the evaluation of simulated monoenergetic images and iodine MD images or iodine maps to improve lesion detection in the

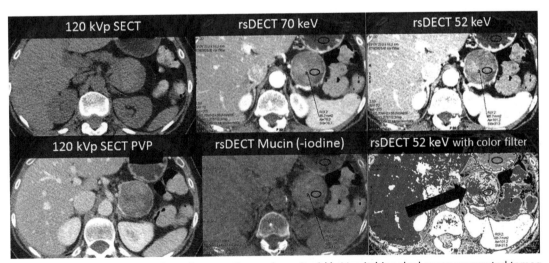

Fig. 5. A 50-year-old woman with mucinous cystic neoplasm. Rapid keV switching dual energy computed tomography image set obtained in the pancreatic parenchymal phase demonstrates the increased depiction of internal septations and nodularity (*arrow*) within this lesion, which contained foci of dysplasia and carcinoma. The type of color overlay or filter may be selected by individual interpreters and saved on the workstation or client server as a standardized protocol, available with a single click.

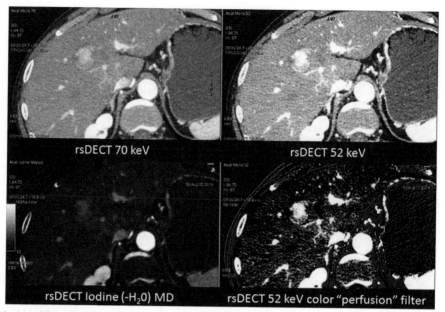

Fig. 6. A 66-year-old man with cirrhosis and a small hepatocellular carcinoma. Rapid keV switching dual energy computed tomography image set obtained in the late hepatic arterial phase demonstrates the increase conspicuity at 52 keV, particularly when the color "perfusion" filter is applied, and both window and level are maintained at the standard 400 W/40L.

liver.[4,32] In a prospective population of 72 patients with 120 small (mean size, 1.7 cm) hypervascular liver lesions scanned in the late arterial phase, 2 independent reviewers measured CNRs at 40, 50, 70, and 77 keV, and in addition subjectively scored lesion conspicuity. The greatest subjective lesion conspicuity and objective measured contrast noise ratios were seen with 50 keV images; however, equal detection of hyperenhancing liver lesions was similar between the 50 and 70 keV images overall.[4] Comparing dual energy iodine measurements with perfusion CT in a prospective trial, Gordic and colleagues[33] showed that at an optimum image acquisition time of 9 seconds after peak threshold in the aorta, the strongest correlations occurred between iodine density and arterial perfusion. Importantly, in a cohort of patients being screened for hepatocellular carcinoma, measurements of estimated radiation exposures including volumetric CT dose index, dose–length product, and size-specific dose estimate were compared between single energy CT and DECT in an intrapatient comparison, and with similar image noise in the liver, all of these parameters were lower for DECT compared with single energy CT.[3]

DECT has been used to better identify iodine in tumor thrombus in patients with hepatocellular carcinoma[34] (**Fig. 7**). Other strategic uses of iodine images available with DECT involve assessment for the effectiveness of locoregional therapies for hepatocellular carcinoma or metastases, including

improved conspicuity of ablation zone margins compared with blended images[35] and in response to transarterial chemoembolization.[36] These iodine images may be enhanced by color coding and, when used, result in decreased uncertainty for the diagnosis of recurrent hepatocellular carcinoma, improved interobserver agreement, and a decrease in interpretation time.[36] Extremely pertinent to the practice of oncology is the detection of small hypovascular metastases in the liver, and although the literature is not robust in this application as yet, using lower keV and iodine MD images holds promise for improved detection (**Fig. 8**). An excellent summary of the use of DECT in the liver as well as other abdominal and pelvic organs is provided in the white papers of the Society of Computed Body Tomography and Magnetic Resonance.[37]

Key points: liver neoplasms

DECT 50 keV simulated monoenergetic images and iodine MD images are used to improve the evaluation of focal hepatic lesions, whether primary or metastatic, and iodine images are helpful in locoregional therapeutic response assessment.

Bowel

The use of DECT may aid in the visualization of hyperenhancing bowel lesions such as carcinoid tumors, both in identification of the primary lesion as well as in evaluation of metastatic disease in the

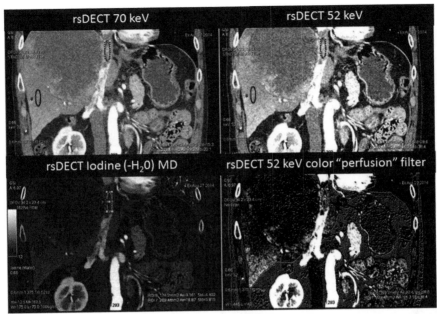

Fig. 7. A 57-year-old man with a large hepatocellular carcinoma and tumor thrombus within the inferior vena cava. Rapid kV switching dual energy computed tomography image set obtained in late hepatic arterial phase shows that the large tumor occupying the majority of the posterior liver has a rim of viable hyperenhancing tissue, but is largely necrotic. The region of interest in the thrombus within the inferior vena cava measures 1.9 mg/mL iodine, indicating enhancement and thus tumoral rather than bland thrombus. This enhancement may also be visualized qualitatively as high signal on the colorized low keV image.

liver (Fig. 9). Cohorts of patients with gastrointestinal stromal tumors have been evaluated with DECT, and work thus far has indicated that the use of monoenergetic images (Fig. 10) provides better image quality than polyenergetic blended images and is less dependent on patient size.[38] DECT is useful to evaluate response in gastrointestinal stromal tumors during therapy with targeted agents, and the change in quantitative iodine content has been found to be a more predictive imaging biomarker of clinical benefit then either anatomic based the Response Evaluation Criteria In Solid Tumors (RECIST) or Choi criteria.[39] The use of colorized low keV and/or iodine map images can help to identify new areas of recurrence in previously treated tumor regions (Fig. 11). Similarly, depiction of the iodine content of hypervascular bowel metastases such as in patients with melanoma is possible (Fig. 12), and can serve as a new biomarker for response to

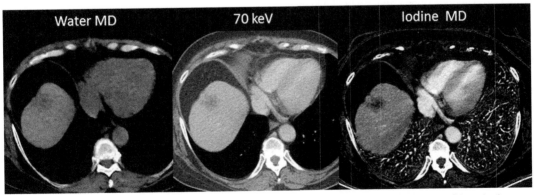

Fig. 8. A 43-year-old man with colorectal carcinoma metastatic to the liver. Rapid kV switching dual energy computed tomography images obtained in portal venous phase demonstrate improved depiction of the margins of the metastasis in the anterior hepatic dome on the iodine material density image compared with the 70 keV or "PACS equivalent" image.

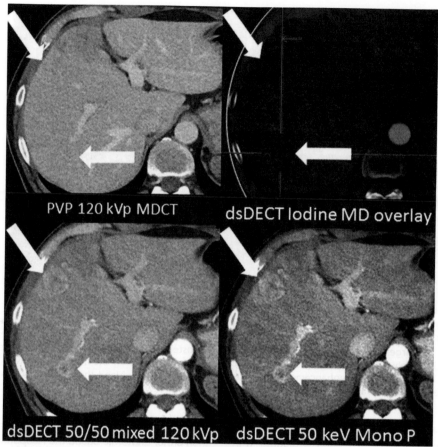

Fig. 9. A 54-year-old man with a carcinoid tumor metastatic to the liver. Dual source dual energy computed tomography image set obtained in the late hepatic arterial phase reveals the iodine overlay (*upper right image*) compared with the blended and monoenergetic plus images for depiction of the hypervascular metastases (*arrows*). The metastases are not seen on the portal venous phase single energy computed tomography.

novel therapies. Much of the more recent work in DECT and bowel neoplasms involves investigation of patients with rectal cancer. Various lesion iodine concentration biomarkers obtained during arterial and/or portal venous phase may be useful in evaluating the degree of tumor differentiation in patients with colon cancer compared with standard imaging.[40,41] Using dual energy to more accurately assess malignant lymph nodes in the mesorectum is an area of active investigation.[42–44] Evaluation of the response to neoadjuvant treatment in patients with locally advanced rectal adenocarcinoma may benefit from DECT techniques, because changes in quantitative image parameters differed significantly after treatment compared with pretreatment values in patients with this disease.[45]

Key points: bowel neoplasms
Lower keV DECT simulated monoenergetic images may aid in the detection of hyperenhancing bowel neoplasms and hepatic metastases, and

quantitative iodine MD images are useful to predict therapeutic response. Rectal carcinoma is an avid area of DECT research at present.

Kidney

The potential value of DECT for evaluation of renal neoplasms was identified early in the trajectory of the clinical use of DECT, with Graser and colleagues[46] suggesting that single phase contrast-enhanced DECT could allow for the characterization of renal masses as benign or malignant. In one of the earliest studies using the dual source DECT technology for a combined phantom and clinical study, iodine concentration was measured with very high accuracy in the phantom. Then in the clinical cohort that followed, papillary renal cell carcinomas (RCCs) demonstrated lower normalized iodine concentration than clear cell types.[47] The first rapid kV switching technology report on 39 subjects with 83 lesions revealed

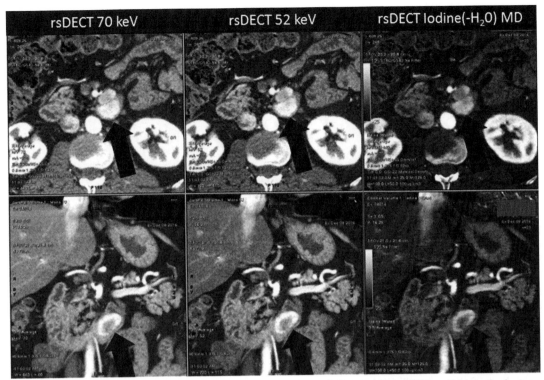

Fig. 10. A 46-year-old man with duodenal gastrointestinal stromal tumor. Rapid kV switching dual energy computed tomography image set obtained during the late hepatic arterial phase reveals a hyperenhancing, focally centrally necrotic lesion (*arrow*) in the fourth portion of the duodenum, without luminal obstruction or extension beyond the serosal surface.

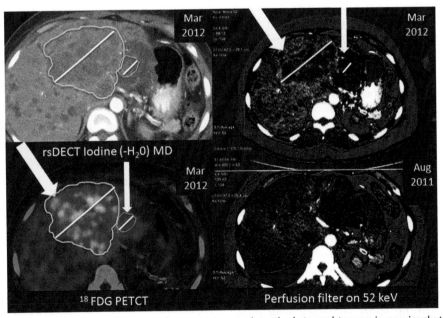

Fig. 11. A 67-year-old woman with new and recurrent gastrointestinal stromal tumors in previously treated hepatic metastatic lesions. Rapid kV switching dual energy computed tomography image set obtained during the late hepatic arterial phase shows the new area of enhancing tumor in the smaller lesion in the lateral segment (*narrow arrow upper right image*) as well as the new medial segment heterogeneously enhancing metastasis (*larger arrow*), compared with the same level 8 months earlier (*lower right*). The PET/computed tomography image (*lower left*) at the same anatomic level shows relative comparison of fluorodeoxyglucose activity to the enhancing component on the iodine material density image.

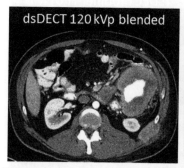
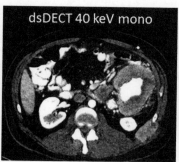
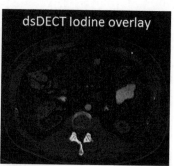

dsDECT 120 kVp blended   **dsDECT 40 keV mono**   **dsDECT Iodine overlay**

Fig. 12. Melanoma metastases to the small bowel and muscle. Dual source dual energy computed tomography image set obtained during the late hepatic arterial phase demonstrates the large jejunal metastasis in the left upper quadrant with excavated bowel lumen, as well as the lesion in the posterolateral abdominal wall. Note that the axial 40 keV monoenergetic plus image has very little noise and excellently depicts the margins of the mass. The color overlay on the iodine image helps to visually demarcate enhancement within the tumor. (*Courtesy of* Anushri Parakh, MD, Massachusetts General Hospital, Boston, MA; with permission.)

that, although the iodine overlay images were sensitive, iodine MD images with quantitative measurement of lesion iodine content was more specific for identification of enhancing versus non-enhancing lesions.[48] In the ensuing years, various reports added to the evidence that DECT techniques provide not only confirmation of enhancement based on Hounsfield unit numbers or tissue iodine content analysis,[49–52] but also could be used to suggest tumor grade[53] or histology.[54] It should be noted that, for many clear cell RCCs, robust and unequivocal enhancement is evident both qualitatively and quantitatively on post contrast-only CT images, whether obtained in arterial (Fig. 13), venous, or nephrographic phase, and whether conventional single energy CT or DECT scanning techniques are used. This is particularly true when the lesion is contour altering, but is also possible when the lesion is small.

However, the real clinical challenge lies in evaluation of lesser enhancing histologic subtypes, such as papillary renal carcinomas or low Fuhrman grade clear cell renal carcinomas compared with complex cysts, and this is where DECT can provide added value to state of the art MDCT practice. Zarzour and colleagues[52] determined with the rapid kV switching technology that the iodine thresholds for discriminating between complex cysts and papillary RCC were lower than the iodine content threshold for discriminating between papillary RCC (Fig. 14), and clear cell RCC (Fig. 15). One caveat that deserves special consideration is that, for lesser enhancing renal neoplasms such as papillary RCCs, the timing of image acquisition must be in the nephrographic or excretory phase to avoid false-negative errors based on iodine quantification. It is very important to note that the various DECT technologies do not measure iodine in the same manner because the

physics behind the image generation and creation are very different.[1,50] Moreover, the magnitude of variance in virtual monoenergetic CT numbers is a function of the selected energy level[55] and lesion iodine content is less accurately measured, particularly at lower concentrations. Therefore, thresholds published in the literature (Table 1) for a certain type of scanner must be abided when applying these values to one's own practice.

DECT is clearly a technology that is gaining traction in the characterization of indeterminate renal masses,[56] and features unique to this

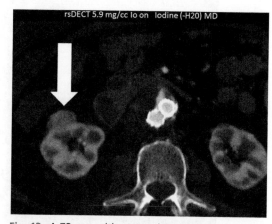

Fig. 13. A 72-year-old man undergoing a dual energy computed tomography angiogram to evaluate aortic endovascular repair. The rapid KV switching iodine (`H$_2$O) material density image obtained during arterial phase 10 s after peak enhancement in the aorta reveals an incidentally detected hyperenhancing mass (*arrow*) projecting anteriorly from the right renal midportion. The lesion contains 5.9 mg/mL iodine and is consistent with a clear cell renal cell carcinoma. An endoleak is also well-depicted on the iodine material density image.

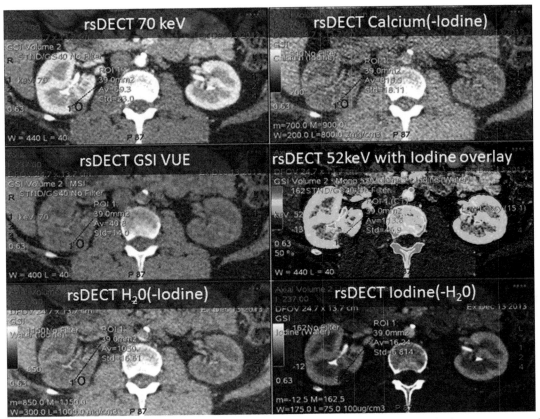

Fig. 14. A 60-year-old man with papillary renal cell carcinoma (RCC). Rapid kV switching dual energy computed tomography image set obtained with the split-bolus technique reveals a very small lesion in the posterior aspect of the right renal midportion, which contains 1.6 mg/mL iodine (*lower right*) and demonstrates an increase in computed tomography (CT) numbers from 41 Hounsfield units (HU) on the virtual unenhanced examination (*middle left*) to 69 HU on the 70 keV image (*upper left*), also confirming enhancement. With both of these methods, neoplasm can be confirmed on a post contrast-only CT, without a dedicated unenhanced acquisition; whereas, if the value of 69 HU was seen on a post contrast-only single energy material density CT image, the differential diagnosis would include a complex (hyperdense) cyst versus a less-enhancing RCC, and a conventional unenhanced image would have to be obtained to determine potential enhancement.

technology, such as virtual monoenergetic imaging to overcome pseudoenhancement of cysts or the use of colorized iodine maps, must be tempered with knowledge of interpretive traps as pointed out herein.[57] Nevertheless, in an important article addressing the clinical conundrum of differentiating between solid versus benign but complex cystic lesions, which may both present as slightly hyperdense focal masses incidentally discovered on a single post-contrast CT scan, iodine overlay images were equivalent to standard precontrast and postcontrast Hounsfield unit enhancement analysis for the identification of enhancement.[58] Using other types of reconstructions such as Z effective images to differentiate benign from malignant lesions has been explored.[59] DECT with iodine material MD quantitative analysis improves specificity for characterization of small renal lesions over conventional attenuation measurements, although the sensitivity is not improved.[60] Finally, characterization of incidentally lesions with DECT can reduce the radiation dose by allowing generation of virtual unenhanced images.[60,61]

Key points: renal neoplasms

The identification of iodine in renal lesions with DECT is equally sensitive and more specific than standard Hounsfield unit number enhancement to identify renal neoplasms, but published thresholds are DECT hardware and software technology dependent and, therefore, should be used with attention to study details; DECT can be used to characterize renal lesions incidentally detected on a single postcontrast abdominal CT scan.

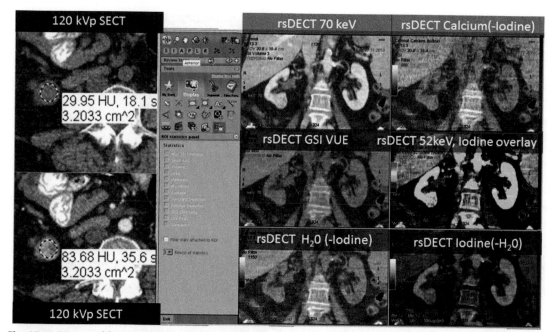

Fig. 15. A 73-year-old woman with clear cell renal cell carcinoma. Rapid kV switching dual energy computed tomography image set obtained in nephrographic phase and reconstructed coronally at 2.5 mm through the level of the right lower pole enhancing mass reveals enhancement using the standard conventional unenhanced and single energy venous phase CT images (*left column*), and the corresponding appearance on the varied dual energy images. The upper middle image represents the "PACS equivalent" image and the lower right the iodine image. In this case the iodine measured 4.97 mg/mL. Note that the CT number within the mass on the virtual unenhanced examination image in the middle center is 30 Hounsfield units, equivalent to the conventional unenhanced value.

Table 1				
Iodine content thresholds for renal mass enhancement				
	Threshold	**System**	**Types of Lesions**	**Accuracy**
Chandarana et al,[47] 2011	Did not calculate	dsDECT	10 cysts, 3 complex cysts, 6 RCC	Not calculated; mean mg/mL "enhancing" lesion 2.12 mg/mL
Kaza et al,[48] 2011	2.0 mg/mL	rsDECT	83 total; 10 "enhancing"	Sens 90, Spec 94, PPV82 NPV 97, Accuracy 94%
Ascenti et al,[50] 2013	0.5 mg/mL	dsDECT	72 total; 18 ccRCC and 5 pRCC	Sens 100, Spec 94, PPV 100, NPV 100, Accuracy 97%
Mileto et al,[51] 2014	0.5 mg/mL	dsDECT	80 total; 17 ccRCC and 6 pRCC	Sens 100, Spec 98, PPV 97, NPV 100
Mileto et al,[53] 2014	0.9 mg/mL (varied with type and grade)	dsDECT	67 ccRCC, 21 pRCC	Accuracy 95%
Zarzour et al,[52] 2016	1.22 (arterial)	rsDECT	46 ccRCC, 27pRCC, 54 complex cysts	Sens 86, Spec 92, PPV 92, NPV 92
	1.28 (nephrographic)			Sens 85, Spec 96, PPV 92, NPV 92

Abbreviations: DECT, dual energy computed tomography; dsDECT, dual source dual energy computed tomography; NPV, negative predictive value; PPV, positive predictive value; RCC, renal cell carcinoma; rsDECT, rapid kV switching dual energy computed tomography; Sens, sensitivity; Spec, specificity.

Adrenal

DECT provides comparable to slightly lower sensitivity for the diagnosis of lipid-rich adenomas than conventional single energy MDCT, but may improve the characterization of lipid-poor adenomas.[62] The earliest evaluations of the use of virtual noncontrast types of DECT images to accurately characterize incidentally discovered adrenal lesions focused on whether the reconstructed images were equivalent to true unenhanced conventional polyenergetic 120 kVp images. This was so the long-standing clinically accepted threshold for benign typical lipid-rich adenomas being 10 Hounsfield units or less could be applied to DECT virtual noncontrast images.[63–65] As explained in other articles, the Hounsfield units produced on virtual noncontrast or virtual unenhanced DECT images are not equivalent to those created with polyenergetic single energy CT at 120 kVp, but in many cases they are sufficiently correlative[66] so that whether using 3 material decomposition virtual noncontrast images with

dual source DECT or using a number of types of virtual unenhanced images on the rapid kV switching technology such as 140 KV, fat (-iodine) or water (-iodine) material decomposition basis pair analysis,[67–69] approximately two-thirds of the time, incidentally discovered adrenal lesions can be characterized as benign lipid-rich adenomas on a postcontrast DECT scan and no further evaluation is required (**Fig. 16**). This is true whether the virtual noncontrast images are crated from unenhanced, arterial, venous, or delayed phase DECT acquisitions.[62,64,70]

Mileto and colleagues[69] were the first to suggest that DECT imaging might be better than conventional unenhanced single energy CT scans in characterizing adrenal lesions after performing a retrospective study of 38 consecutive patients with 47 adrenal nodules and discovering that DECT MD measurements using fat (-iodine) and fat (-H_2O) material decomposition basis pairs could differentiate adenomas from nonadenomas with a specificity of 100%. Furthermore, these unique images provided improved identification

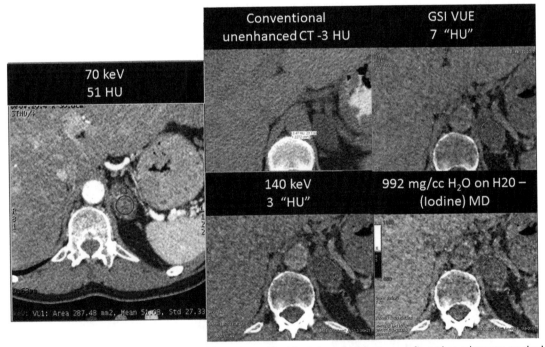

Fig. 16. A 54-year-old man with a carcinoid tumor and incidental adrenal lesion confirmed as adenoma on dual energy computed tomography (DECT). Rapid kV switching DECT image set obtained in late hepatic arterial phase (patient being scanned for potential carcinoid metastases) demonstrates a value of 7 Hounsfield units on the virtual unenhanced examination. This image is a material suppression iodine image generated in projection space through a voxel-based multimodality decomposition converted to a monoenergetic 70 keV image. Other forms of virtual unenhanced images include a 140 keV image, with iodine still apparent but moving the energy furthest away from the K edge of iodine (33.2 keV) and thus reducing the effect of iodine on signal within the image, and a water (-iodine) material decomposition image. Note that the Hounsfield units obtained with the various dual-energy images are not equivalent to the conventional unenhanced image value, but are adequate for confirming adenoma.

of lipid-poor adenomas over standard unenhanced multidetector CT scans. Others have investigated focal adrenal lesions in novel ways including applying DECT to washout during dedicated adrenal imaging,[71] or using other reconstructions such as z effective images.[72]

Key points: adrenal lesions

Much of the work in adrenal DECT scanning has been to address the problem of incidentally discovered masses, and the majority of the time, benign lesions can be confirmed on a single postcontrast DECT scan and obviate the need for further imaging.

Gynecologic Tumors

The body of work that has been performed thus far in the evaluation of gynecologic malignancies with DECT scans is small, but the principles and proven advantages for the evaluation of soft tissue tumors elsewhere in the abdomen apply for these types of soft tissue tumors as well. Specific research in ovarian, cervical, and endometrial cancer has been performed. DECT has the potential to improve diagnostic performance, specifically to differentiate between simple cystic lesions and primary ovarian cancer,[73] much in the same way that complexity in pancreatic cystic lesions can be optimally visualized with lower keV images or enhancement in nodules can be confirmed with quantitative iodine analysis. A retrospective study comparing DECT imaging features with endovaginal ultrasound examination in a cohort of 39

patients with endometrial carcinoma revealed that 50 keV images used to predict deep myometrial invasion had the highest correlation with surgical findings, iodine MD images and endovaginal ultrasound diagnostic performance were equivalent and next best, and 70 kV images performed least optimally.[74] And, in the context of using DECT image biomarkers as predictors of therapeutic response, Jiang and colleagues[75] found that compared with RECIST 1.0, higher arterial phase quantitative normalized iodine content on pretreatment DECT predicted favorable response.

Key points: gynecologic neoplasms

Early studies suggest benefits for lower keV and iodine MD reconstructions for the optimal viewing of ovarian and endometrial cancers, and quantitative iodine content may be useful in predicting response to therapy in patients with cervical cancer.

Pulmonary

DECT applications in the chest have the potential to add functional assessment as well as improved visualization or characterization of lesions as benign (inflammatory or infectious) or malignant. Like other soft tissue tumors, DECT imaging biomarkers may help to predict the biologic activity or response of tumors. As far as the type of images used to evaluate pulmonary neoplasms, iodine images can help to delineate tumor from surrounding collapsed lung (**Fig. 17**). Simulated monoenergetic images reconstructed at 40 keV monoenergetic

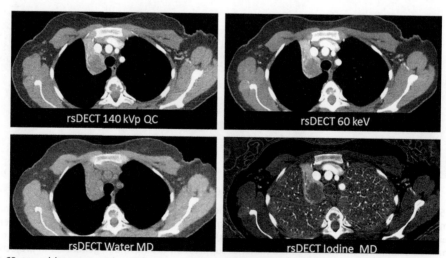

Fig. 17. A 62-year-old woman with a right paratracheal mass. Rapid kV switching dual energy computed tomography image set demonstrates a 140 kVp quality control image (*upper left*), which is provided to rapidly assess the area of scan coverage immediately after acquisition during image reconstruction but is also available for diagnostic interpretation. Compare the increased conspicuity of the hypoenhancing central tumor clearly delineated from the adjacent enhancing collapsed lung parenchyma, particularly well-seen on the iodine material density image in the lower right. (*Courtesy of* Anushri Parakh, MD, Massachusetts General Hospital, Boston, MA; with permission.)

plus provided the highest tumor CNR; however, readers preferred to view 55 keV monoenergetic plus images for overall image quality and tumor delineation.[76] This finding is similar to optimal viewing energies for abdominal neoplasms.

For the evaluation of an isolated pulmonary nodule, the identification of calcification using virtual noncontrast images may be of benefit,[77] and various DECT methods of quantitative iodine evaluation might help to determine etiologies. In a retrospective study of 139 patients with histologic confirmation, early and late phase DECT normalized iodine concentrations differentiated lesions into active inflammation (highest normalized iodine content), malignancy (mid-range iodine content), and tuberculosis (lowest normalized iodine content).[78] Quantitative analysis using iodine maps in addition to the identification of uniformity within a ground glass nodular lesion produced an increased ability to predict the presence of invasive adenocarcinoma versus noninvasive or minimally invasive adenocarcinomas compared with virtual noncontrast imaging[79] (**Fig. 18**). For the evaluation of larger lesions, DECT iodine concentration, normalized iodine concentration, and slope of spectral attenuation help to distinguish between malignant pulmonary masses and inflammatory masses.[80] However, other studies failed to demonstrate iodine quantification methods that separated pulmonary lesions into benign or malignant etiologies.[81] For the evaluation of lymph nodes, quantitative iodine content may help to discriminate metastatic and benign lymph nodes in lung cancer just as in rectal cancer. In a population of 61 patients with non–small cell lung cancer confirmed pathologically, a sensitivity of 80%, specificity of 65%, and accuracy of 73% were recorded when a threshold of 29.32×100 μg/cm^3 and 0.4328 represented the iodine content and normalized iodine content values, respectively.[82]

Pulmonary function after surgical resection in patients with lung cancer may be evaluated with DECT scanning using volumetric iodine values to observe not only perfusion but also lung volumes.[83] Quantitative iodine uptake parameters obtained at peak arterial enhancement in patients with lung cancer correlated with perfusion parameters calculated by first past dual input perfusion CT,[84] and there is active investigation on the usefulness of quantitative iodine in pulmonary neoplasms, with mixed initial results. Iodine quantification parameters could not distinguish between adenocarcinoma and squamous cell carcinoma in a population of 61 patients with pathologic confirmation.[82] However, other studies have shown positive results that may depend on the timing of the image acquisition relative to contrast administration. For example, Iwano and colleagues[85] showed that the volumetric iodine content of lung cancers was significantly associated with the degree of differentiation, in that high-grade tumors tended to have lower iodine volumes than low-grade tumors in a cohort of 60 patients. Iodine content derived from DECT acquisitions at 2 and 3 minute delays positively correlated with immunostaining scores of hypoxia-inducible factor 1 alpha but not vascular endothelial growth factor or epidermal growth factor recptor.[86] In a cohort of 48 patients with non–small cell lung cancer, quantitative biomarkers differed in patients whose specimens revealed positive expression of vascular endothelial growth factor and negative/moderately expressed vascular endothelial growth factor.[87] This is an area for DECT application that warrants further study.

Finally, iodine uptake may help to predict response in lung cancer. In a population of 31 patients with non–small cell lung cancer who had DECT scans before and at a mean of 8 weeks after anti-epidermal growth factor receptor therapy, arterial and venous phase acquisition iodine

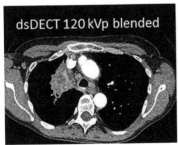 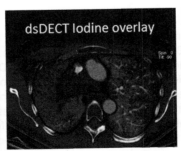 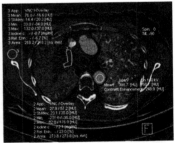

Fig. 18. Right upper lobe lung cancer. Dual source dual energy computed tomography image set reveals a heterogeneous right upper lobe mass on the blended image (*left image*) as well as the iodine overlay images, which depict the degree of enhancement qualitatively (*center*) and may also be interrogated with a freehand region of interest for quantitative iodine content measurement (*right*). (*Courtesy of* Anushri Parakh, MD, Massachusetts General Hospital, Boston, MA; with permission.)

analysis revealed a significant decrease in iodine uptake in the venous phase in responders. In addition, a prototype imaging biomarker the authors called arterial enhancement fraction was significantly different between pretreatment and post-treatment tumor assessment for responders versus nonresponders.[88] In summary, lower energy simulated monoenergetic reconstructions and iodine imaging are useful for pulmonary neoplasm detection, but the clinical application of quantitative iodine values remains an exciting area of research. More information about pulmonary applications of DECT scans can be found in the white papers of the Society of Computed Body Tomography and Magnetic Resonance.[89]

Key points: pulmonary neoplasms
DECT applications in the chest have the potential to add functional assessment as well as improved visualization or characterization of tumors, with use of lower keV and iodine image reconstructions used now for routine clinical viewing, and quantitative iodine for individual tumor tissue specific analysis and response prediction remaining in the research realm at present.

Head and Neck Cancers

There are several reviews focused on DECT scanning in patients with squamous cell carcinoma of the head and neck, and emerging applications include improved lesion visualization as well as determination of tumor extent and evaluation of critical anatomic structures.[90] The optimum lower KV energy level for viewing of squamous head and neck cancer is 60 keV.[91] In addition, a reduction in metal artifacts using dual energy techniques can aid in overall improved visualization and evaluation.[92] As in other soft tissue tumors, color-coded iodine maps are used to increase lesion detection visually and are particularly helpful for the improved depiction of cartilage invasion by hypopharyngeal and laryngeal squamous cell carcinoma,[93] as well as nodal involvement.[94] Previous evaluations of dual source DECT systems have demonstrated that the percentage and method of image blending of the 80 and 140 kVp datasets affects CNRs and, thus, the visualization of complex head and neck tumors. More recently, Scholtz and associations[95] suggested that subjective overall imaging quality was improved with nonlinear compared with linear blending techniques. Linear blending applies only to dual source DECT scans. In the future, the viewing of simulated monoenergetic images available on all types of major DECT scanners may be preferred if noise correction techniques improve for the head and neck region, much as they are now preferred for

all soft tissue tumor evaluations in the abdomen. In a recent study directly comparing 40 keV simulated monoenergetic images with single energy CT scans in a cohort of 60 patients with head and neck squamous cell carcinoma, the lower keV images demonstrated very high interreader agreement and improved tumor visibility based on objective image data measurements; in addition, the 40 keV images were preferred by readers whether they were subspecialty trained or general radiologists.[96]

Key points: head and neck cancers
If using a dual source DECT scanner, nonlinear blending is helpful for improved image quality. The use of lower keV simulated monoenergetic images and iodine overlay images increases detection of tumors and visualization of important surrounding structures on all systems, and DECT metal artifact reduction techniques may also contribute to improved visualization of this complex anatomy.

Miscellaneous Tumors

Other soft tissue tumors including melanoma and lymphoma have been preliminarily investigated with DECT applications, specifically the use of iodine MD images for markedly improved detection of intramuscular melanoma metastases[97] (see **Fig. 12**) and for assessment of melanoma metastasis response to targeted therapy.[98] The use of quantitative iodine metrics for response in lymphoma patients[99] has also been investigated. However, there is scant evidence in the literature to make recommendations for routine clinical DECT viewing best practices at this time. One additional exciting area of dual energy is the ability to perform calcium subtractions to evaluate bone marrow. This may be useful not only in musculoskeletal lesions, but also may be helpful in the evaluation of patients with multiple myeloma spectrum.[100]

SUMMARY

Key take-home points for evaluation of oncologic patients with DECT revolve around the use of lower energy (low keV) reconstructed images and iodine MD images. Lower keV simulated monoenergetic images optimize tumor to nontumoral attenuation differences and increase CNRs to improve lesion detection. Iodine images are helpful from a qualitative standpoint for image interpretation because they result in improved detection and characterization of tumors, and from a quantitative assessment approach to interrogate specific properties of tissues and predict/assess therapeutic response. Iodine thresholds for confirmation of enhancement depend on the type of dual energy system used, and this must be taken into consideration when implementing these modalities in clinical practice. The largest body of knowledge involves abdominal neoplasms, and not only can DECT benefit patients with renal, pancreas, and liver (primary and metastatic) lesions, it can help to solve clinical conundrums of incidentally discovered adrenal nodules and hyperdense cysts first identified on CTs obtained in a postcontrast setting, obviating the need to obtain additional imaging. This reduces excess radiation required for a true noncontrast series, reduces costs, and relieves anxiety of further testing on the part of the patient. In the future, reducing the intravenous iodinated contrast dose coupled with lower keV imaging may prove the real strength and added value of DECT in the evaluation of patients with neoplasms.

REFERENCES

1. Foley WD, Shuman WP, Siegel MJ, et al. White paper of the SCBT-MR on DECT, part 2: radiation dose and iodine sensitivity. J Comput Assist Tomogr 2016;40(6):846–50.

2. Uhrig M, Simons D, Kachelrieß M, et al. Advanced abdominal imaging with DECT is feasible without increasing radiation dose. Cancer Imaging 2016; 16(1):15.

3. Purysko AS, Primak AN, Baker ME, et al. Comparison of radiation dose and image quality from single-energy and dual-energy CT examinations in the same patients screened for hepatocellular carcinoma. Clin Radiol 2014;69(12): e538–44.

4. Shuman WP, Green DE, Busey JM. Dual-energy liver CT: effect of monochromatic imaging on lesion detection, conspicuity, and contrast-to-noise ratio of hypervascular lesions on late arterial phase. AJR Am J Roentgenol 2014;203(3):601–6.

5. Cramer TW, Fletcher JG, Paden RG, et al. A primer on the use of dual-energy CT in the evaluation of commonly encountered neoplasms. Abdom Radiol (NY) 2016;41(8):1618–31.

6. Thaiss WM, Sauter AW, Bongers M, et al. Clinical applications for DECT versus dynamic contrast enhanced CT in oncology. Eur J Radiol 2015; 84(12):2368–79.

7. Thaiss WM, Haberland U, Kaufmann S, et al. Iodine concentration as a perfusion surrogate marker in oncology: further elucidation of the underlying mechanisms using Volume Perfusion CT with 80 kVp. Eur Radiol 2016;26(9):2929–36.

8. Stiller W, Skornitzke S, Fritz F, et al. Correlation of quantitative dual-energy computed tomography iodine maps and abdominal computed tomography perfusion measurements: are single-acquisition dual-energy computed tomography iodine maps more than a reduced-dose surrogate of conventional computed tomography perfusion? Invest Radiol 2015;50(10):703–8.

9. Knobloch G, Jost G, Huppertz A, et al. Dual-energy computed tomography for the assessment of early treatment effects of regorafenib in a preclinical tumor model: comparison with dynamic contrast-enhanced CT and conventional contrast-enhanced single-energy CT. Eur Radiol 2014; 24(8):1896–905.

10. Chung YE, You JS, Lee HJ, et al. Possible contrast media reduction with low keV monoenergetic images in the detection of focal liver lesions: a dual-energy CT animal study. PLoS One 2015;10(7): e0133170.

11. Husarik DB, Gordic S, Desbiolles L, et al. Advanced virtual monoenergetic computed tomography of hyperattenuating and hypoattenuating liver lesions: ex-vivo and patient experience in various body sizes. Invest Radiol 2015;50(10): 695–702.

12. Paul J, Vogl TJ, Mbalisike EC. Oncological applications of dual-energy computed tomography imaging. J Comput Assist Tomogr 2014;38(6):834–42.

13. Siegel MJ, Kaza RK, Bolus DV, et al. White paper of the SCBT-MR on DECT, part 1: technology and terminology. J Comput Assist Tomogr 2016;40(6): 841–5.

14. Macari M, Spieler B, Kim D, et al. Dual-source dual-energy MDCT of pancreatic adenocarcinoma: initial observations with data generated at 80 kVp and at simulated weighted-average 120 kVp. AJR Am J Roentgenol 2010;194:W27–32.

15. Patel BN, Thomas JV, Lockhart ME, et al. Single-source dual-energy spectral multidetector CT of pancreatic adenocarcinoma: optimization of energy level viewing significantly increases lesion contrast. Clin Radiol 2013;68(2):148–54.

16. McNamara MM, Little MD, Alexander LF, et al. Multireader evaluation of lesion conspicuity in small pancreatic adenocarcinomas: complimentary value of iodine MD and low keV simulated monoenergetic images using multiphasic rapid kVp-switching DECT. Abdom Imaging 2015;40(5): 1230–40.

17. Gupta S, Wagner-Bartak N, Jensen CT, et al. Dual-energy CT of pancreatic adenocarcinoma: reproducibility of primary tumor measurements and assessment of tumor conspicuity and margin sharpness. Abdom Radiol (NY) 2016;41(7):1317–24.

18. Bhosale P, Le O, Balachandran A, et al. Quantitative and qualitative comparison of single-source dual-energy computed tomography and 120-kVp computed tomography for the assessment of

pancreatic ductal adenocarcinoma. J Comput Assist Tomogr 2015;39(6):907–13.

19. Hardie AD, Picard MM, Camp ER, et al. Application of an advanced image-based virtual monoenergetic reconstruction of dual source dual-energy CT Data at low keV increases image quality for routine pancreas imaging. J Comput Assist Tomogr 2015;39(5):716–20.

20. Frellesen C, Fessler F, Hardie AD, et al. Dual-energy CT of the pancreas: improved carcinoma-to-pancreas contrast with a noise-optimized monoenergetic reconstruction algorithm. Eur J Radiol 2015;84(11):2052–8.

21. Quiney B, Harris A, McLaughlin P, et al. Dual-energy CT increases reader confidence in the detection and diagnosis of hypoattenuating pancreatic lesions. Abdom Imaging 2015;40(4):859–64.

22. Brook OR, Gourtsoyianni S, Brook A, et al. Split-bolus spectral multidetector CT of the pancreas: assessment of radiation dose and tumor conspicuity. Radiology 2013;269(1):139–48.

23. Noid G, Schott D, Chen X, et al. Enhancement of CT-texture based treatment response detection for pancreatic cancer using dual-energy CT. AAPM 2017,SU-F-FS4–2. Available at: http://www.aapm.org/meetings/2017AM/PRAbs.asp?mid=127&aid=36625. Accessed September 30, 2017.

24. Morgan DE. DECT of the abdomen. Abdom Imaging 2014;39:108–34.

25. Lin XZ, Wu ZY, Tao R, et al. Dual energy spectral CT imaging of insulinoma-Value in preoperative diagnosis compared with conventional multidetector CT. Eur J Radiol 2012;81(10):2487–94.

26. Yin Q, Zou X, Zai X, et al. Pancreatic ductal adenocarcinoma and chronic mass-forming pancreatitis: differentiation with dual-energy MDCT in spectral imaging mode. Eur J Radiol 2015;84(12):2470–6.

27. Marin D, Nelson RC, Ehsan S, et al. Hypervascular liver tumors: low tube voltage, high tube current multidetector CT during late hepatic arterial phase for detection—initial clinical experience. Radiology 2009;251:771–9.

28. Park JH, Kim SH, Park HS, et al. Added value of 80 kVp images to averaged 120 kVp images in the detection of hepatocellular carcinomas in liver transplantation candidates using dual-source dual-energy MDCT: results of JAFROC analysis. Eur J Radiol 2011;80:e76–85.

29. Lv P, Lin XZ, Li J, et al. Differentiation of small hepatic hemangioma from small hepatocellular carcinoma: recently introduced spectral CT method. Radiology 2011;259:720–9.

30. Lv P, Lin XZ, Chen K, et al. Spectral CT in patients with small HCC: investigation of image quality and diagnostic accuracy. Eur Radiol 2012;22:2117.

31. Anzidei M, Di Martino M, Sacconi B, et al. Evaluation of image quality, radiation dose and diagnostic performance of dual-energy CT datasets in patients with hepatocellular carcinoma. Clin Radiol 2015;70(9):966–73.

32. Caruso D, De Cecco CN, Schoepf UJ, et al. Can dual-energy computed tomography improve visualization of hypoenhancing liver lesions in portal venous phase? Assessment of advanced image-based virtual monoenergetic images. Clin Imaging 2017;41:118–24.

33. Gordic S, Puippe GD, Krauss B, et al. Correlation between dual-energy and perfusion CT in patients with hepatocellular carcinoma. Radiology 2016; 280(1):78–87.

34. Ascenti G, Sofia C, Mazziotti S, et al. Dual-energy CT with iodine quantification in distinguishing between bland and neoplastic portal vein thrombosis in patients with hepatocellular carcinoma. Clin Radiol 2016;71(9):938.e1-9.

35. Lee SH, Lee JM, Kim KW, et al. Dual-energy computed tomography to assess tumor response to hepatic radiofrequency ablation. Invest Radiol 2011;46(2):77–84.

36. Lee JA, Jeong WK, Kim Y, et al. Dual-energy CT to detect recurrent HCC after TACE: initial experience of color-coded iodine CT imaging. Eur J Radiol 2013;82(4):569–76.

37. De Cecco CN, Boll DT, Bolus DN, et al. White paper of the SCBT-MR on DECT, part 4: abdominal and pelvic applications. J Comput Assist Tomogr 2017;41(1):8–14.

38. Sudarski S, Apfaltrer P, Nance JW, et al. Objective and subjective image quality of liver parenchyma and hepatic metastases with virtual monoenergetic dual-source dual-energy CT reconstructions: an analysis in patients with gastrointestinal stromal tumor. Acad Radiol 2014;21(4):514–22.

39. Meyer M, Hohenberger P, Apfaltrer P, et al. CT-based response assessment of advanced gastrointestinal stromal tumor: DECT provides a more predictive imaging biomarker of clinical benefit than RECIST or Choi criteria. Eur J Radiol 2013; 82(6):923–8.

40. Chuang-Bo Y, Tai-Ping H, Hai-Feng D, et al. Quantitative assessment of the degree of differentiation in colon cancer with dual-energy spectral CT. Abdom Radiol (NY) 2017;42(11):2591–6.

41. Gong HX, Zhang KB, Wu LM, et al. Dual energy spectral CT imaging for colorectal cancer grading: a preliminary study. PLoS One 2016;11(2): e0147756.

42. Al-Najami I, Beets-Tan RG, Madsen G, et al. Dual-energy CT of rectal cancer specimens: a CT-based method for mesorectal lymph node characterization. Dis Colon Rectum 2016;59(7):640–7.

43. Kato T, Uehara K, Ishigaki S, et al. Clinical significance of dual-energy CT-derived iodine

quantification in the diagnosis of metastatic LN in colorectal cancer. Eur J Surg Oncol 2015; 41(11):1464–70.

44. Liu H, Yan F, Pan Z, et al. Evaluation of dual energy spectral CT in differentiating metastatic from non-metastatic lymph nodes in rectal cancer: initial experience. Eur J Radiol 2015;84(2): 228–34.

45. Al-Najami I, Drue HC, Steele R, et al. DECT - a possible new method to assess regression of rectal cancers after neoadjuvant treatment. J Surg Oncol 2017;116(8):984–8.

46. Graser A, Becker CR, Staehler M, et al. Single-phase dual-energy CT allows for characterization of renal masses as benign or malignant. Invest Radiol 2010;45(7):399–405.

47. Chandarana H, Megibow AJ, Cohen BA, et al. Iodine quantification with dual-energy CT: phantom study and preliminary experience with renal masses. AJR Am J Roentgenol 2011;196(6):W693–700.

48. Kaza RK, Caoili EM, Cohan RH, et al. Distinguishing enhancing from nonenhancing renal lesions with fast kilovoltage-switching dual-energy CT. AJR Am J Roentgenol 2011;197:1375–81.

49. Neville AM, Gupta RJ, Miller CM, et al. Detection of renal lesion enhancement with dual-energy multidetector CT. Radiology 2011;259(1):173–83.

50. Ascenti G, Mazziotti S, Mileto A, et al. Dual-source dual-energy CT evaluation of complex cystic renal masses. AJR Am J Roentgenology 2012;199: 1026–34.

51. Mileto A, Marin D, Ramirez-Giraldo JC, et al. Accuracy of contrast-enhanced dual-energy MDCT for the assessment of iodine uptake in renal lesions. Am J Roentgenology 2014;202: W466–74.

52. Zarzour JG, Milner D, Valentin R, et al. Quantitative iodine content threshold for discrimination of papillary renal cell carcinomas from complex cysts using rapid kV-switching DECT. Abdom Radiol 2017;42(3):727–34.

53. Mileto A, Marin D, Alfaro-Cordoba M, et al. Iodine quantification to distinguish clear cell from papillary renal cell carcinoma at dual-energy multidetector CT: a multireader diagnostic performance study. Radiology 2014;273(3):813–20.

54. Dai C, Cao Y, Jia Y, et al. Differentiation of renal cell carcinoma subtypes with different iodine quantification methods using single-phase contrast-enhanced dual-energy CT: areal vs. volumetric analyses. Abdom Radiol (NY) 2018;43(3):672–8.

55. Mileto A, Barina A, Marin, et al. Virtual monochromatic images from dual-energy multidetector CT: variance in CT numbers from the same lesion between single-source projection-based and dual-source image-based implementations. Radiology 2016;(279):269–77.

56. Heilbrun ME, Remer EM, Casalino DD, et al. ACR appropriateness criteria indeterminate renal mass. J Am Coll Radiol 2015;12(4):333–41.

57. Mileto A, Sofue K, Marin D. Imaging the renal lesion with dual-energy multidetector CT and multi-energy applications in clinical practice: what can it truly do for you? Eur Radiol 2016;26(10):3677–90.

58. Cha D, Kim CK, Park JJ, et al. Evaluation of hyperdense renal lesions incidentally detected on single-phase post-contrast CT using dual-energy CT. Br J Radiol 2016;89(1062):20150860.

59. Mileto A, Allen BC, Pietryga JA, et al. Characterization of incidental renal mass with dual-energy CT: diagnostic accuracy of effective atomic number maps for discriminating nonenhancing cysts from enhancing masses. Am J Roentgenology 2017; 209:W221–30.

60. Marin D, Davis D, Choudhury K, et al. Characterization of small focal renal lesions: diagnostic accuracy with single-phase contrast-enhanced dual-energy CT with material attenuation analysis compared with conventional attenuation measurements. Radiology 2017;284(3):737–47.

61. Kaza RK, Ananthakrishnan L, Kambadakone A, et al. Update of dual-energy CT applications in the genitourinary tract. AJR Am J Roentgenol 2017;208(6):1185–92.

62. Schieda N, Siegelman ES. Update on CT and MRI of adrenal nodules. AJR Am J Roentgenol 2017; 208(6):1206–17.

63. Gnannt R, Fisher M, Goetti R, et al. AJR 2011: dual-energy CT for characterization of the incidental adrenal mass: preliminary observations. AJR Am J Roentgenol 2012;198(1):138–44.

64. Ho LM, Marin D, Neville AM, et al. Characterization of adrenal nodules with dual-energy CT: can virtual unenhanced attenuation values replace true unenhanced attenuation values? Am J Roentgenology 2012;198:840–5.

65. Helck A, Hummel N, Meinel FG, et al. Can single-phase dual-energy CT reliably identify adrenal adenomas? Eur Radiol 2014;24(7):1636–42.

66. Slebocki K, Kraus B, Chang DH, et al. Incidental findings in abdominal dual-energy computed tomography: correlation between true noncontrast and virtual noncontrast images considering renal and liver cysts and adrenal masses. J Comput Assist Tomogr 2017;41(2):294–7.

67. Morgan DE, Weber A, Lockhart ME, et al. Differentiation of high lipid-content from low lipid content adrenal lesions using single source rapid kVp-switching dual energy multidetector CT. J Comput Assist Tomogr 2013;37(6):937–43.

68. Glazer DI, Maturen KE, Kaza RK, et al. Adrenal Incidentaloma triage with single-source (fast-kilovoltage switch) dual-energy CT. AJR Am J Roentgenol 2014;203(2):329–35.

69. Mileto A, Nelson RC, Marin D, et al. Dual-energy multidetector CT for the characterization of incidental adrenal nodules: diagnostic performance of contrast-enhanced material density analysis. Radiology 2015;274:445–54.

70. Botsikas D, Triponez F, Boudabbous S, et al. Incidental adrenal lesions detected on enhanced abdominal dual-energy CT: can the diagnostic workup be shortened by the implementation of virtual unenhanced images? Eur J Radiol 2014; 83(10):1746–51.

71. Kim YK, Park BK, Kim CK, et al. Adenoma characterization: adrenal protocol with dual-energy CT. Radiology 2013;267(1):155–63.

72. Ju Y, Liu A, Dong Y, et al. The value of nonenhanced single-source dual-energy CT for differentiating metastases from adenoma in adrenal glands. Acad Radiol 2015;22(7):834–9.

73. Benveniste AP, de Castro Faria S, Broering G, et al. Potential application of dual-energy CT in gynecologic cancer: initial experience. AJR Am J Roentgenol 2017;208(3):695–705.

74. Rizzo S, Femia M, Radice D, et al. Evaluation of deep myometrial invasion in endometrial cancer patients: is dual-energy CT an option? Radiol Med 2018;123(1):13–9.

75. Jiang C, Yang P, Lei J, et al. The application of iodine quantitative information obtained by dual-source dual-energy computed tomography on chemoradiotherapy effect monitoring for cervical cancer: a preliminary study. J Comput Assist Tomogr 2017;41(5):737–45.

76. Frellesen C, Kaup M, Wichmann JL, et al. Noise-optimized advanced image-based virtual monoenergetic imaging for improved visualization of lung cancer: comparison with traditional virtual monoenergetic imaging. Eur J Radiol 2016;85(3): 665–72.

77. Chae EJ, Song JW, Krauss B, et al. Dual-energy computed tomography characterization of solid pulmonary nodules. J Thorac Imaging 2010;25(4): 301–10.

78. Lin JZ, Zhang L, Zhang CY, et al. Application of gemstone spectral computed tomography imaging in the characterization of solitary pulmonary nodules: preliminary result. J Comput Assist Tomogr 2016;40(6):907–11.

79. Son JY, Lee HY, Kim JH, et al. Quantitative CT analysis of pulmonary ground-glass opacity nodules for distinguishing invasive adenocarcinoma from non-invasive or minimally invasive adenocarcinoma: the added value of using iodine mapping. Eur Radiol 2016;26(1):43–54.

80. Hou WS, Wu HW, Yin Y, et al. Differentiation of lung cancers from inflammatory masses with dual-energy spectral CT imaging. Acad Radiol 2015; 22(3):337–44.

81. González-Pérez V, Arana E, Barrios M, et al. Differentiation of benign and malignant lung lesions: dual-energy computed tomography findings. Eur J Radiol 2016;85(10):1765–72.

82. Li X, Meng X, Ye Z. Iodine quantification to characterize primary lesions, metastatic and non-metastatic lymph nodes in lung cancers by dual energy computed tomography: an initial experience. Eur J Radiol 2016;85(6):1219–23.

83. Choe J, Lee SM, Chae EJ, et al. Evaluation of postoperative lung volume and perfusion changes by dual-energy computed tomography in patients with lung cancer. Eur J Radiol 2017; 90:166–73.

84. Chen X, Xu Y, Duan J, et al. Correlation of iodine uptake and perfusion parameters between dual-energy CT imaging and first-pass dual-input perfusion CT in lung cancer. Medicine (Baltimore) 2017; 96(28):e7479.

85. Iwano S, Ito R, Umakoshi H, et al. Evaluation of lung cancer by enhanced dual-energy CT: association between three-dimensional iodine concentration and tumour differentiation. Br J Radiol 2015; 88(1055):20150224.

86. Yanagawa M, Morii E, Hata A, et al. Dual-energy dynamic CT of lung adenocarcinoma: correlation of iodine uptake with tumor gene expression. Eur J Radiol 2016;85(8):1407–13.

87. Li GJ, Gao J, Wang GL, et al. Correlation between vascular endothelial growth factor and quantitative dual-energy spectral CT in non-small-cell lung cancer. Clin Radiol 2016;71(4):363–8.

88. Baxa J, Matouskova T, Krakorova G, et al. Dual-phase dual-energy CT in patients treated with erlotinib for advanced non-small cell lung cancer: possible benefits of iodine quantification in response assessment. Eur Radiol 2016;26(8): 2828–36.

89. DeCecco CN, Schoepf UJ, Steinbach L, et al. White paper of the SCBT-MR on DECT, part 3: vascular, cardiac, pulmonary and musculoskeletal applications. J Comput Assist Tomogr 2017;41(1): 1–7.

90. Forghani R, Kelly HR, Curtin HD. Applications of dual-energy computed tomography for the evaluation of head and neck squamous cell carcinoma. Neuroimaging Clin N Am 2017;27(3):445–59.

91. Albrecht MH, Scholtz JE, Kraft J, et al. Assessment of an advanced monoenergetic reconstruction technique in dual-energy computed tomography of head and neck cancer. Eur Radiol 2015;25(8): 2493–501.

92. Lam S, Gupta R, Kelly H, et al. Multiparametric evaluation of head and neck squamous cell carcinoma using a single-source dual-energy CT with fast kVp switching: state of the art. Cancers (Basel) 2015;7(4):2201–16.

93. Kuno H, Onaya H, Iwafa R, et al. Evaluation of cartilage invasion by laryngeal and hypopharyngeal squamous cell carcinoma with dual-energy CT. Radiology 2012;265:488–96.

94. Tawfik AM, Razek AA, Kerl JM, et al. Comparison of dual-energy CT-derived iodine content and iodine overlay of normal, inflammatory, and metastatic squamous cell carcinoma cervical lymph nodes. Eur Radiol 2014;24(3):574–80.

95. Scholtz JE, Hüsers K, Kaup M, et al. Non-linear image blending improves visualization of head and neck primary squamous cell carcinoma compared to linear blending in dual-energy CT. Clin Radiol 2015;70(2):168–75.

96. Forghani R, Kelly H, Yu E, et al. Low-energy virtual monochromatic dual-energy computed tomography images for the evaluation of head and neck squamous cell carcinoma: a study of tumor visibility compared with single-energy computed tomography and user acceptance. J Comput Assist Tomogr 2017;41(4):565–71.

97. Uhrig M, Simons D, Bonekamp D, et al. Improved detection of melanoma metastases by iodine maps from DECT. Eur J Radiol 2017;90:27–33.

98. Uhrig M, Simons D, Ganten MK, et al. Histogram analysis of iodine maps from dual energy computed tomography for monitoring targeted therapy of melanoma patients. Future Oncol 2015;11(4):591–606.

99. Kulkarni NM, Pinho DF, Narayanan S, et al. Imaging for oncologic response assessment in lymphoma. AJR Am J Roentgenol 2017;208(1):18–31.

100. Thomas C, Schabel C, Krauss B, et al. Dual-energy CT: virtual calcium subtraction for assessment of bone marrow involvement of the spine in multiple myeloma. AJR Am J Roentgenol 2015;204(3): W324–31.

Advanced Musculoskeletal Applications of Dual-Energy Computed Tomography

William D. Wong, BSC*, Samad Shah, MD,
Nicolas Murray, MD, Frances Walstra, MD, Faisal Khosa, MD,
Savvas Nicolaou, MD

KEYWORDS

- Dual-energy CT • Musculoskeletal • Gout • Bone marrow edema • Artifact reduction • Tendons
- Ligaments

KEY POINTS

- Dual-energy computed tomography (DECT) is a well-established tool for the detection of gout. Its noninvasive nature and the ability to evaluate the spine, periarticular tissues, tendons, and ligaments make it especially useful.
- The detection of bone marrow edema with the DECT virtual noncalcium technique provides an alternative to MR imaging and can improve the identification of subtle fractures.
- The DECT virtual monochromatic image simulates a CT image resulting from a single-energy source and can thus mitigate beam-hardening artifacts.
- DECT's ability to highlight collagen renders it capable of assessing tendon, ligament, and intervertebral disc pathologic states.
- Upcoming applications of DECT include arthrography, calculation of bone mineral density, and the evaluation of other inflammatory arthropathies, musculoskeletal infections, and skeletal metastases.

INTRODUCTION

The musculoskeletal (MSK) system paints a unique picture in radiology because it combines 2 very different domains of anatomy: bones and soft tissues. This dichotomy of MSK composition has confined imaging with the tradeoff between optimal osseous and soft tissue detail. The premier modalities for analysis of these 2 major anatomic domains emerged as computed tomography (CT) and MR imaging. CT provides excellent bony detail and fast acquisition times. MR imaging, on the other hand, is considered the gold standard for soft tissue imaging; however, it is slower to obtain and harbors contraindications such as metallic implants.

Dual-energy CT (DECT) has presented itself as the technology that can combine some of the capabilities of MR imaging with those of CT, along with some powerful, additional benefits. Although it first became clinically available in 2005,[1] its theoretic inception dates back to the late 1970s when X-ray spectra of different energies were shown to elicit different tissue signatures.[2,3]

The purpose of this article is to update radiologists on the current status of DECT research and

Disclosure Statement: Dr F. Khosa is the recipient of the Canadian Association of Radiologists Leadership Scholarship (2017) and the Vancouver Coastal Leadership Award (2017). The authors have no other relevant disclosures. There was no commercial funding for this study.
Department of Radiology, Vancouver General Hospital, 899 West 12th Avenue, Vancouver, BC V5Z1M9, Canada
* Corresponding author.
E-mail address: b.wong22@alumni.ubc.ca

Radiol Clin N Am 56 (2018) 587–600
https://doi.org/10.1016/j.rcl.2018.03.003
0033-8389/18/© 2018 Elsevier Inc. All rights reserved.

to provide context in the form of relevant clinical cases.

INFLAMMATORY ARTHRITIS
Gout

DECT has a growing role in the diagnosis of inflammatory arthritis, most notably in gout (**Figs. 1** and **2**). Gout, characterized by monosodium urate (MSU) crystal deposition, is the most prevalent crystal arthropathy, found to affect nearly 4% of Americans in 2007.[4] It is a painful condition associated with cardiovascular disease and accompanying risk factors, holding a 1.26 relative risk for cardiovascular death.[5] Beyond the classic presentation of gout in the first metatarsophalangeal joint, Mallinson and colleagues[6] outlined the most common locations. Out of 148 subjects with gout, 68% had it in the foot, 56% in the knee, 53% in the ankle, and 28% in the elbow. Clinically, gout may be confused with septic arthritis, osteoarthritis, pseudogout, rheumatoid arthritis, or tumors.[7]

Literature from 2009 to 2017 suggests that DECT has a 90% to 100% sensitivity and an 83% to 89% specificity for diagnosing gout.[8] However, gout tends to reveal itself most clearly in chronic, tophaceous forms of the disease; in these cases, imaging would not be clinically indicated. In 2015, a study by Bongartz and colleagues[9] showed DECT to have a sensitivity of 90% and specificity of 83% for diagnosing gout in 40 subjects with gout and 41 with other articular diseases; subjects with a history of tophaceous gout were excluded from this study, which makes it more relevant to early disease. Nevertheless, the study noted that all of its false negatives stemmed from subjects in the first 6 weeks of their first flare of gout.[9]

The noninvasive nature of DECT makes it a promising tool in the workup of atypical presentations of gout and tracking of treatment success by quantitative volumetric measurements.[10] DECT has been used to detect MSU crystal deposition in periarticular tissues,[11] tendons, and ligaments (**Fig. 3**).[12] DECT has been able to detect gout in the spine, which models situations in which joints may be inaccessible or there is lack of sufficient joint fluid for analysis.[13]

A limitation is that accuracy may be reduced in early disease, especially in the first 6 weeks of an initial flare.[9] Common contributors to false-positive assessments for gout on DECT include osteoarthritis[9] and nail bed or skin artifacts.[14]

Pseudogout

DECT may also have potential for evaluating other crystal arthropathies, such as pseudogout. A case of pseudogout has been described in which calcium pyrophosphate accumulation mimicked tophaceous gout in the distal radioulnar joint. DECT identified calcium deposition in the absence of MSU crystals.[15] Pseudogout can be suggested by findings on ultrasound or MR imaging but usually requires radiographic evidence of calcified deposits and final confirmation of calcium pyrophosphate crystals in synovial fluid.[16] DECT offers additional information in this context through its ability to distinguish between crystal types noninvasively.

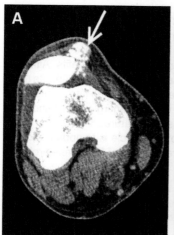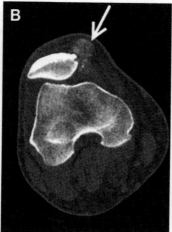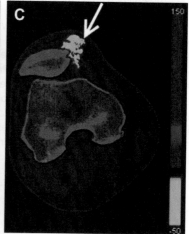

Fig. 1. A 56-year-old man presenting with a soft tissue mass of the knee and a history of trauma. Initial radiographs were unremarkable. Soft tissue kernel (*A*) and bone kernel (*B*) CT images reveal a mineralized mass (*arrows*) with mild erosions suggestive of posttraumatic heterotopic calcifications, pigmented villonodular synovitis, or gout. (*C*) DECT clearly visualizes monosodium urate crystals (*green*).

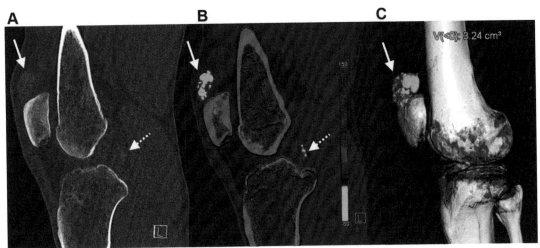

Fig. 2. A 54-year-old man presenting with a suprapatellar mass. (*A*) A large mass with faint internal calcifications is noted superior to the patella (*arrows*). Mineralization is also noted posterior to the articulation (*dotted arrow*). (*B*, *C*) On the DECT urate detection application, the lesion contains a large proportion of MSU, color-coded in green, in keeping with gout tophus. The second area of calcification also corresponds to soft tissue MSU deposition (*dotted arrow*).

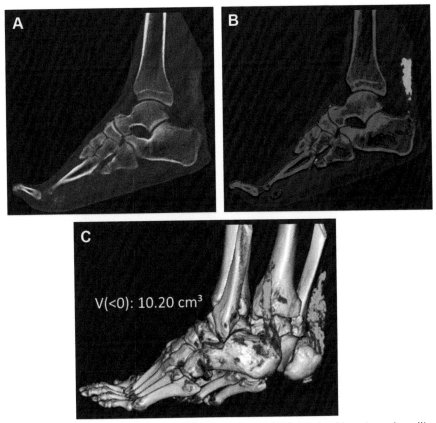

Fig. 3. A 52-year-old patient with a history of gout presenting with bilateral ankle pain and swelling. (*A*) CT depicts mineralization in the Achilles tendon (right ankle). (*B*) DECT identifies mineralization as monosodium urate crystals (*green*). (*C*) DECT quantitative volumetric measurements of MSU crystal deposition may assist in management.

Other Inflammatory Arthropathies

Recently, DECT has been put forth as a potential tool for assessing other types of inflammatory arthritis, including septic, rheumatoid, and psoriatic arthritis.[17–19] In a prospective study of 16 psoriasis subjects with finger joint symptoms, Fukuda and colleagues[18] endorsed a sensitivity of 78% and a specificity of 87% for inflammatory lesions (synovitis, flexor tenosynovitis, and periarticular inflammation), which was the same as contrast-enhanced MR imaging for all lesions except for synovitis. They discussed how MR imaging remained superior for the detection of inflammatory lesions; however, DECT was better able to assess structural changes (erosion and proliferation), which was significant as proliferation is a key finding in psoriatic arthritis.

Further research is needed to define DECT's capabilities in the evaluation of inflammatory arthropathies other than gout.

BONE MARROW EDEMA

Bone marrow edema (BME) can be the result of hemorrhage in the bone marrow related to trauma[20] or can be related to infections, tumors, or avascular necrosis in a nontraumatic setting (Figs. 4–6). The gold standard for BME detection is MR imaging, in which BME results in reduced signal on T1-weighted images and increased signal on fat-suppressed T2 images due to the increase in water concentration. However, MR imaging's dependence on the homogeneity of the magnetic field can result in incomplete fat saturation mimicking BME; this issue does not exist with DECT.[19] Furthermore, due to its fast acquisition times and ability to outline fine cortical detail, CT is usually the first line in the emergency trauma setting.[21]

The DECT virtual noncalcium (VNCa) technique was introduced by Pache and colleagues[22] in 2010. Using the absorption profiles of bone mineral, yellow marrow, and red marrow over the 2 DECT X-ray spectra, this method allows for calcium subtraction through image postprocessing.[22] The VNCa image allows for color mapping over a CT image for targeted assessment of BME. DECT VNCa has been shown to be a sensitive and specific tool for BME detection (Table 1). Use of DECT would allow additional information to be obtained immediately in the emergency department; namely, in assisting the detection of subtle fractures. It may also serve as a convenient alternative modality to MR imaging when MR imaging is contraindicated or not easily accessed.

Vertebral Compression Fractures

The utility for DECT in the diagnosis of vertebral compression fractures is a promising clinical application. Vertebral compression fractures are a significant cause of morbidity and mortality, and are underdiagnosed in clinical practice.[31] There is a rising push for the use of imaging in the detection of vertebral fractures by radiologists.[32] Osteoporotic bone is often problematic in the evaluation by traditional CT because fractures may not be well-defined.[28] Thus, the accompanying presence of BME may aid in fracture detection.

Wang and colleagues[24] found a cutoff of −80 HU (using the VNCa technique) to identify edematous vertebral bodies with compression fractures with 96% sensitivity and 98% specificity in vertebral bodies with less than 50% sclerosis and/or air. The VNCa technique has the potential to decrease referrals for MR imaging by 36% to 87% (between a less experienced vs an experienced reader) for the diagnosis of thoracolumbar vertebral fractures.[28]

Hip Fractures

Hip fractures are another age-related pathologic condition that may present an application for DECT. DECT has been used to detect radiographically occult hip fractures with 90% sensitivity and 40% specificity. False positives were mainly due to degenerative changes appearing as BME, which represents a limitation of DECT VNCa.[33] The presence of BME was found in 83% of occult hip fractures.[33] Recently, DECT has been shown to increase sensitivity by 4% to 5% when used in addition to bone reconstruction images compared with the reconstructions on their own.[30]

Limitations

A limitation of DECT VNCa is that it is unable to evaluate BME in the immediate vicinity to cortical bone due to confusion with the cortex.[22] Proximity to sclerotic bone or gas may result in artifacts.[23,24] Wang and colleagues[24] noted that these effects restricted their ability to assess vertebral bodies with a height less than 4 mm. Also, interpretation of color-coded VNCa images may take considerable experience to master, which is evident in the variation in results among readers found by Kaup and colleagues.[28]

METAL ARTIFACT REDUCTION

DECT stands as the leading technology for metal artifact reduction in the MSK system without increased radiation exposure.[34] Beam hardening occurs when more low-energy photons are

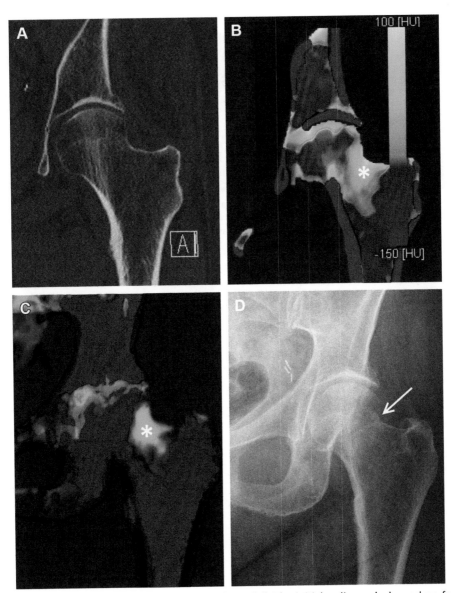

Fig. 4. A 75-year-old man presenting with hip pain after a fall. The initial radiograph showed no fracture but owing to the high clinical suspicion of posttraumatic injury, DECT was performed. (*A*) The CT image notes minimal sclerosis in the femur neck but no clear fracture or cortical disruption. (*B, C*) Bone marrow analysis by DECT notes BME (*asterisks*) of the lateral femur neck due to a fracture. This was confirmed by bone scintigraphy. (*D*) The radiograph performed 2 days posttrauma reveals the posttraumatic sclerosis of a healing fracture (*arrow*).

absorbed than high-energy photons, resulting in a higher energy spectrum of exiting photons. It produces hypoattenuation around dense materials.[34] Attempts to decrease artifacts on multidetector CT include reducing the collimation and pitch of the detector, increasing the energy peak and tube charge, and use of various postprocessing algorithms calibrated to phantoms.[35] These, however, may result in increased radiation dose.[35]

DECT uses 2 polychromatic X-ray sources with different spectra. By combining this dual input in image postprocessing techniques, beam-hardening artifacts can be reduced by producing virtual monochromatic images (**Fig. 7**). A virtual monochromatic image is the linear combination of the 2 CT images, which represents an image that would be the result of a single-energy level photon source.[35] Increasing energies of virtual monoenergetic images beyond 60 keV have been associated with reduced beam-hardening artifacts, with the optimum energies ranging from 108 and 149 keV. Rapid-switching,[35–37] dual-source,[38–42] and dual-layer systems[43] have been successful. Bamberg and colleagues[38]

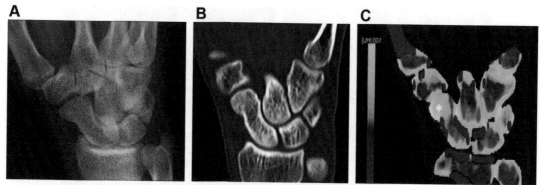

Fig. 5. A 20-year-old woman presenting with wrist pain after a bicycle accident. (*A*) Radiograph notes an irregularity in the body of the scaphoid, suggesting a fracture or nutrient foramen. (*B*) Conventional CT and (*C*) DECT identify a fracture of the scaphoid tubercle with BME clearly visible on DECT (*asterisk*). The absence of a fracture of the scaphoid body improved the prognosis.

imaged 31 subjects with metallic implants with DECT. Image quality and diagnostic value scores were shown to improve by about 49% and 44%, respectively. The density of artifacts decreased from −882 to −341 HU.

Beam-hardening artifact reduction has been shown to improve visualization of the prosthesis and periprosthetic bone, and soft tissues in a variety of prosthesis types.[37] Caution was advised, however, in the evaluation of titanium implants because these did not respond as well as other materials in the artifact reduction software.

Meinel and colleagues[42] found that increasing extrapolated photon energy from 64 to 120 keV decreased artifact severity from 8.0 to 2.0 (*P*<.001) and streak intensity from 871 to 153 HU (*P*<.001) using an approach optimized on a hip phantom and tested on 22 adults with metallic implants for MSK indications. They found ideal parameters to be energy settings at 140 and 100 kilovolt (peak) with a tin filter, tube current ratio

3:1, collimation 32 times 0.6 mm, and pitch of 0.5 at a rotation time of 0.5 seconds per rotation.

TENDONS, LIGAMENTS, AND JOINTS

MR imaging is the gold standard for the evaluation of tendons and ligaments, most commonly performed in the knee.[44] Conventional CT has been shown to be able to identify tendons and ligaments; however, fine detail may be limited due to beam-hardening artifacts.[45] DECT may provide an alternative through its ability to highlight collagen (**Figs. 8** and **9**). Furthermore, DECT arthrography may potentially be used in surgical planning. Conventional CT lacks the capability to produce 3-dimensional reconstructions because it cannot distinguish iodine contrast from nearby bone.[46]

In 2007, Johnson and colleagues[47] demonstrated that DECT was able to highlight collagen by material differentiation, suggesting its application for the

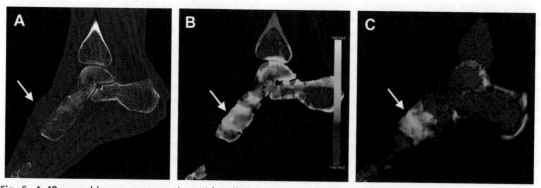

Fig. 6. A 48-year-old woman presenting with cellulitis and skin ulceration on the dorsum on the foot. (*A*) Soft tissue swelling and thickening overlying the medial cuneiform is seen but no definite osseous abnormality is present on the conventional bone reformats. (*B*, *C*) Using DECT bone marrow analysis, widespread signal abnormality is noted throughout the medial cuneiform, likely representing underlying osteomyelitis (*arrows*).

Table 1
Diagnostic performance of dual-energy computed tomography virtual noncalcium for the detection of bone marrow edema compared with MR imaging as the reference standard

	Region	Number of Subjects	Sensitivity (%)	Specificity (%)
Pache et al,[22] 2010	(Knee)	21		
	Femur		79	98
	Tibia		95	92
Guggenberger et al,[23] 2012	Ankle	30	90	81
Wang et al,[24] 2013	Vertebrae (<50% sclerosis and/or air)	63	96	98
Bierry et al,[25] 2014	Vertebrae	20	84	97
Cao et al,[26] 2015	(Knee)	32		
	Femur		74	99
	Tibia		91	100
Karaca et al,[27] 2016	Vertebrae	23	89	99
Kaup et al,[28] 2016	Vertebrae	49	82–94	77–96
Diekhoff et al,[29] 2017	Vertebrae	9	88	100
Kellock et al,[30] 2017	Hip	118	71–91	92–99

Ranges of sensitivity and specificity values represent results from multiple readers.

imaging of tendons and ligaments. In 2008, Sun and colleagues[48] demonstrated DECT's use in ligamentous structures. They scanned 12 subjects with DECT and were able to visualize the partial ligaments in the knee: the patellar, fibular collateral, posterior cruciate, and anterior cruciate ligament (ACL). However, the transversal ligaments, including the lateral and medial patellar retinaculum,

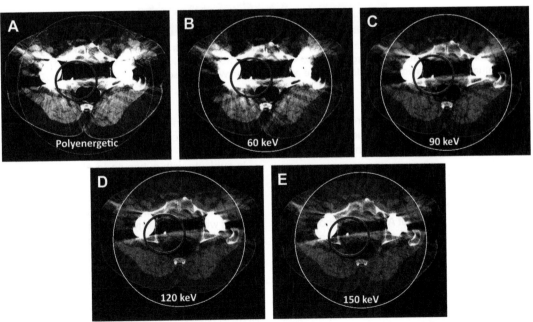

Fig. 7. A 65-year-old man presenting with intermittent right-sided flank pain radiating toward the right scrotum. (A) Bilateral hip prostheses produced severe metal artifacts in the pelvic area that obscure the obstructive renal calculus in the right distal ureter (blue circles) on the conventional polyenergetic image. DECT monoenergetic analysis at (B) 60 keV, (C) 90 keV, (D) 120 keV, and (E) 150 keV demonstrate reduction of artifacts with increasing energy level.

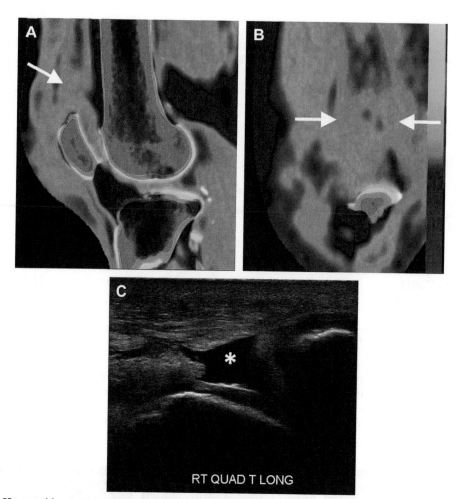

Fig. 8. A 63-year-old man presenting after a fall. (*A*, *B*) DECT analysis shows a complete rupture of the right quadriceps tendon, demonstrated by a large area lacking collagen fibers superior to the patella (*arrows*). (*C*) Ultrasound evaluation confirmed the tendon rupture and retraction with an associated fluid-filled gap (*asterisk*).

and the posterior ligament, were not well visualized.[48] In 2009, Deng and colleagues[49] described DECT's ability to clearly visualize most hand and foot tendons.

DECT has been compared with MR imaging assessment of ACL lesions in porcine models. Both DECT and MR imaging visualized the ACL in 100% of cases. For intact ACLs, both modalities had a 67% sensitivity; MR imaging had a higher specificity (79%) than DECT (71%). In complete ACL tears, DECT had a 75% sensitivity and 69% specificity, whereas MR imaging had a 100% sensitivity and 75% specificity. For anteromedial and posterolateral lesions, both DECT and MR imaging had a much lower sensitivity.[50]

Peltola and Koskinen[51] assessed 18 subjects with acute knee trauma and found DECT to have a 79% sensitivity and 100% specificity for detecting ACL tears. They noted that gemstone

spectral imaging performed better than bone removal and collagen-specific color mapping protocols.

In subjects with subacute to chronic traumatic ACL disruption confirmed by MR imaging, receiver operating characteristic (ROC) curve analysis of DECT performance showed that sagittal oblique images with dual-energy bone removal, soft tissue windowing, and single-energy bone removal were most accurate, with area under the curve (AUC) of 0.95, 0.94, and 0.93, respectively.[52]

Dual-Energy Computed Tomography Arthrography

Chai and colleagues[53] were able to subtract a 25% iodinated contrast mixture from DECT arthrography in 4 out of 12 pig cadaver joints to produce additional virtual unenhanced images.

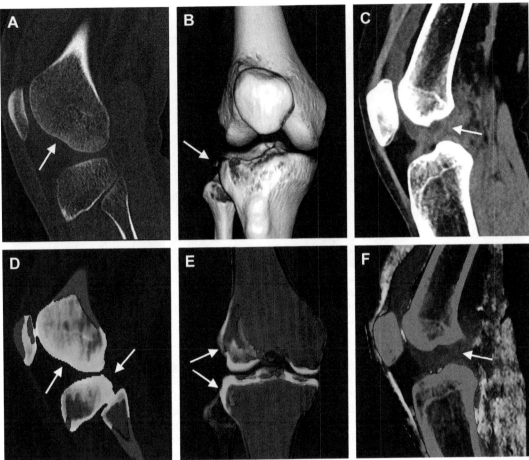

Fig. 9. A 22-year-old woman presenting after a twisting injury. Conventional CT images in (*A*) sagittal bone window and (*B*) 3-dimensional reformat demonstrate a subchondral fracture of the lateral femoral condyle and a Segond fracture of the lateral tibial plateau (*arrows*). (*C*) Evaluation of the cruciate ligaments is limited by conventional CT; heterogeneity is noted in the expected location of the anterior cruciate ligament (ACL), raising the possibility of a tear. (*D, E*) On DECT analysis, BME is present in the lateral femoral condyle and posterior tibia, in keeping with a pivot shift injury. (*F*) DECT demonstrates the absence of collagen fibers in the ACL location, confirming a complete ACL tear.

For arthrography performed on a shoulder phantom, DECT has demonstrated the ability to reduce beam-hardening artifacts and separate contrast from cortical bone.[54] DECT use in arthrography, however, is complicated by the anatomy of the joint. There are 4 materials present in arthrography (bone, soft tissue, synovial fluid, and iodine), and DECT's 3-material decomposition method thus encounters difficulty. Moreover, cartilage is usually the focus of analysis, which may be challenging to assess on DECT due to artifacts produced by adjacent cortical bone.[55]

The literature on the use of DECT in the evaluation of collagenous structures is still developing. As a further avenue for exploration, Murray and colleagues[56] have suggested that DECT using collagen postprocessing techniques may increase diagnostic confidence in assessing disc bulging and herniation. There is potential for the evaluation of degenerative disc disease by DECT (**Fig. 10**). DECT arthrography may aid surgeons in preoperative planning after it is validated in human subjects. Further studies will be needed to render DECT a widespread clinical tool in these domains.

ONCOLOGY

The evaluation of bone metastases is a growing application of DECT, particularly in the evaluation of spinal lesions in oncologic patients (**Table 2**).[56] Kraus and colleagues[57] found that monoenergetic reconstructions of contrast-enhanced portal-venous images significantly improved image

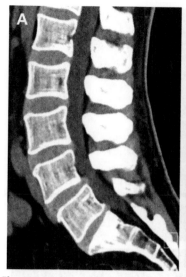 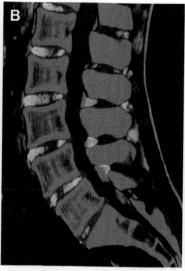 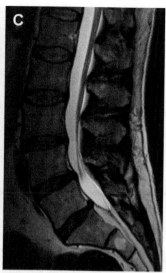

Fig. 10. A 54-year-old man patient presenting with back pain. (*A*) Conventional CT images demonstrate mild disc bulging and disc space narrowing involving the last 3 levels. (*B*) On DECT, early degenerative disc disease is noted, with decreased amount of collagen tissue in the discs. (*C*) MR imaging confirmed this with decreased T2 signal intensity.

quality and identification of spinal metastases in 26 oncologic subjects compared with linearly blended DECT images. The highest contrast to noise ratio was found at 40 keV (on a 5-point scale: conspicuity 4.5 ± 0.7, delineation 4.3 ± 0.9, sharpness 4.2 ± 0.8, confidence 4.6 ± 0.6).

Gemstone DECT has demonstrated a 90% sensitivity and 88% specificity for the differentiation of bone metastases from Schmorl nodes; this distinction is possible due to the higher water content and lower bone content in osteolytic metastases.[58] In subjects with lung cancer, a cutoff value of 68.6 HU on virtual monochromatic spectral imaging had a 93% sensitivity and 93% specificity for distinguishing between osteoblastic metastases and bone islands.[59]

DECT may aid in the detection of bone marrow lesions associated with multiple myeloma (**Fig. 11**). Thomas and colleagues[60] used conventional CT and DECT to assess bone lesions in multiple myeloma, with MR imaging as the reference standard. In 32 multiple myeloma subjects, they found that DECT allowed for the discrimination of pathologic from normal bone marrow with an 89% specificity and 85% specificity compared with MR imaging. They described their study as a proof on concept, however, because DECT performed better than conventional CT for nonlytic lesions but worse for lytic lesions.

Table 2
Potential avenues for dual-energy computed tomography evaluation of metastases

Application	Mechanism	Clinical Use
Quantitative tissue decomposition	Malignant infiltration results in osteolysis and fatty marrow replacement by soft tissue with associated increased vascularity[46]	Differentiation of malignant lesions from Schmorl nodes
Qualitative tissue decomposition	Color-coding or subtraction of bone to highlight abnormal soft tissue[46]	Identification of subtle metastases
Virtual noncontrast images and iodine mapping	Enhancement of malignant soft tissue in lytic lesions[46]	Phasic contrast-enhanced imaging in cancer staging; assessment of nonspecific lucencies

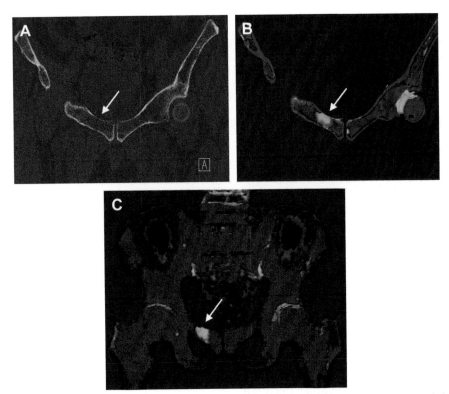

Fig. 11. A 58-year-old man known to have multiple myeloma. (*A*) On conventional CT images, a subtle lucency is noted in the right superior pubic ramus with minimal endosteal scalloping (*arrows*). (*B, C*) This is better shown on DECT analysis using the bone marrow application.

BONE MINERAL DENSITY

DECT's ability to separate materials suggests its use in measuring bone mineral density (BMD), which may be useful for predicting osteoporotic fractures, as well as for surgical assessment.[61,62] With growing elderly populations, osteoporosis and other age-related conditions are becoming an increasing concern. It is estimated that between 2005 and 2025, osteoporosis-related fractures and associated costs will increase by nearly 50% in the United States.[63]

In addition to the diagnosis of vertebral compression fractures and hip fractures discussed earlier, DECT may play a role in osteoporosis assessment through the measurement of BMD. Dual-energy X-ray absorptiometry (DXA) scans are the current standard for BMD measurement.[64] However, DXA produces a 2-dimensional average over the vertebral body, which subjects it to inaccuracies related to variation in volume[65] and soft tissue contributions.[66,67] Quantitative CT has been suggested as an alternative; however, it relies on individual phantom calibration and an increased effective radiation dose.[68,69] DECT might be superior to conventional CT in its ability

to reduce artifacts without additional radiation dose. Furthermore, material decomposition algorithms could allow for isolation and quantification of true bone mineral content.[70] BMD information could conceivably be calculated from abdominal DECT scans to reduce imaging costs.[71]

Wichmann and colleagues[72] compared BMD measurements by DXA and DECT in the lumbar spine and found the measurements to have no statistical correlation. They emphasized how DECT is capable of measuring the true volumetric BMD of the trabecular bone, whereas DXA measurements represent both cortical and trabecular bone. In addition, DECT's ability to minimize artifacts makes it advantageous in measuring BMD around prostheses. Periprosthetic bone loss is thought to be a potential contributor to failure of total hip arthroplasty.[62] In a study of porcine hip specimens, BMD measurements adjacent to acetabular cups were more precise when obtained by DECT than by conventional CT.[62]

There is insufficient literature at this time to validate DECT as a clinical tool for BMD. Nevertheless, it is a promising technique that may find numerous applications.

SUMMARY

DECT is rapidly establishing itself as a valuable tool in MSK imaging. There is substantial evidence for its clinical use in

- Gout
- BME
- Artifact reduction.

The body of DECT literature is small, but promising for

- Tendons and ligaments
- Psoriatic arthritis
- Bone metastases
- Multiple myeloma
- BMD measurement
- Arthrography.

Finally, DECT has been proposed as a potential modality for the evaluation of

- Intervertebral discs
- Rheumatoid arthritis
- Pseudogout
- MSK infections.

A plethora of future innovations await. DECT is a paragon of conceptual physics transformed into an advanced clinical tool. As such, the authors expect that DECT will continue to paint new strokes of color on the horizon of MSK imaging.

REFERENCES

1. Flohr TG, McCollough CH, Bruder H, et al. First performance evaluation of a dual-source CT (DSCT) system. Eur Radiol 2006;16(2):256–68.
2. Di Chiro G, Brooks RA, Kessler RM, et al. Tissue signatures with dual-energy computed tomography. Radiology 1979;131(2):521–3.
3. Millner MR, McDavid WD, Waggener RG, et al. Physics: extraction of information from CT scans at different energies. J Comput Assist Tomogr 1979;3(4):579.
4. Zhu Y, Pandya BJ, Choi HK. Prevalence of gout and hyperuricemia in the US general population: the National Health and Nutrition Examination Survey 2007-2008: prevalence of gout and hyperuricemia in the US. Arthritis Rheum 2011;63(10):3136–41.
5. Roddy E, Doherty M. Gout. Epidemiology of gout. Arthritis Res Ther 2010;12(6):223.
6. Mallinson PI, Reagan AC, Coupal T, et al. The distribution of urate deposition within the extremities in gout: a review of 148 dual-energy CT cases. Skeletal Radiol 2014;43(3):277–81.
7. Chou H, Chin TY, Peh WCG. Dual-energy CT in gout - A review of current concepts and applications. J Med Radiat Sci 2017;64(1):41–51.
8. Rech HJ, Cavallaro A. Dual-energy-computertomographie-Diagnostik bei Gicht. Z Rheumatol 2017; 76(7):580–8.
9. Bongartz T, Glazebrook KN, Kavros SJ, et al. Dual-energy CT for the diagnosis of gout: an accuracy and diagnostic yield study. Ann Rheum Dis 2015; 74(6):1072–7.
10. Desai MA, Peterson JJ, Garner HW, et al. Clinical utility of dual-energy CT for evaluation of tophaceous gout. Radiographics 2011;31(5):1365–75.
11. Glazebrook KN, Guimarães LS, Murthy NS, et al. Identification of intraarticular and periarticular uric acid crystals with dual-energy CT: initial evaluation. Radiology 2011;261(2):516–24.
12. Dalbeth N, Kalluru R, Aati O, et al. Tendon involvement in the feet of patients with gout: a dual-energy CT study. Ann Rheum Dis 2013;72(9):1545–8.
13. Parikh P, Butendieck R, Kransdorf M, et al. Detection of lumbar facet joint gouty arthritis using dual-energy computed tomography. J Rheumatol 2010; 37(10):2190–1.
14. Mallinson PI, Coupal T, Reisinger C, et al. Artifacts in dual-energy CT gout protocol: a review of 50 suspected cases with an artifact identification guide. Am J Roentgenol 2014;203(1):W103–9.
15. Ward IM, Scott JN, Mansfield LT, et al. Dual-energy computed tomography demonstrating destructive calcium pyrophosphate deposition disease of the distal radioulnar joint mimicking tophaceous gout. J Clin Rheumatol 2015;21(6):314–7.
16. Soldatos T, Pezeshk P, Ezzati F, et al. Cross-sectional imaging of adult crystal and inflammatory arthropathies. Skeletal Radiol 2016;45(9):1173–91.
17. Fukuda T, Umezawa Y, Asahina A, et al. Dual energy CT iodine map for delineating inflammation of inflammatory arthritis. Eur Radiol 2017;27(12): 5034–40.
18. Fukuda T, Umezawa Y, Tojo S, et al. Initial experience of using dual-energy CT with an iodine overlay image for hand psoriatic arthritis: comparison study with contrast-enhanced MR imaging. Radiology 2017;284(1):134–42.
19. Diekhoff T, Scheel M, Hermann S, et al. Osteitis: a retrospective feasibility study comparing single-source dual-energy CT to MRI in selected patients with suspected acute gout. Skeletal Radiol 2017; 46(2):185–90.
20. Thiryayi WA, Thiryayi SA, Freemont AJ. Histopathological perspective on bone marrow oedema, reactive bone change and haemorrhage. Eur J Radiol 2008;67(1):62–7.
21. Memarsadeghi M, Breitenseher MJ, Schaefer-Prokop C, et al. Occult scaphoid fractures: comparison of multidetector CT and MR imaging—initial experience. Radiology 2006;240(1):169–76.
22. Pache G, Krauss B, Strohm P, et al. Dual-energy CT virtual noncalcium technique: detecting posttraumatic

bone marrow lesions—feasibility study. Radiology 2010;256(2):617–24.

23. Guggenberger R, Gnannt R, Hodler J, et al. Diagnostic performance of dual-energy CT for the detection of traumatic bone marrow lesions in the ankle: comparison with MR imaging. Radiology 2012; 264(1):164–73.

24. Wang C-K, Tsai J-M, Chuang M-T, et al. Bone marrow edema in vertebral compression fractures: detection with dual-energy CT. Radiology 2013; 269(2):525–33.

25. Bierry G, Venkatasamy A, Kremer S, et al. Dual-energy CT in vertebral compression fractures: performance of visual and quantitative analysis for bone marrow edema demonstration with comparison to MRI. Skeletal Radiol 2014;43(4):485–92.

26. Cao J, Wang Y, Kong X, et al. Good interrater reliability of a new grading system in detecting traumatic bone marrow lesions in the knee by dual energy CT virtual non-calcium images. Eur J Radiol 2015;84(6):1109–15.

27. Karaca L, Yuceler Z, Kantarci M, et al. The feasibility of dual-energy CT in differentiation of vertebral compression fractures. Br J Radiol 2016;89(1057): 20150300.

28. Kaup M, Wichmann JL, Scholtz J-E, et al. Dual-energy CT–based display of bone marrow edema in osteoporotic vertebral compression fractures: impact on diagnostic accuracy of radiologists with varying levels of experience in correlation to MR imaging. Radiology 2016;280(2):510–9.

29. Diekhoff T, Hermann KG, Pumberger M, et al. Dual-energy CT virtual non-calcium technique for detection of bone marrow edema in patients with vertebral fractures: a prospective feasibility study on a single- source volume CT scanner. Eur J Radiol 2017;87:59–65.

30. Kellock TT, Nicolaou S, Kim SSY, et al. Detection of bone marrow edema in nondisplaced hip fractures: utility of a virtual noncalcium dual-energy CT application. Radiology 2017;284(3):798–805.

31. Papaioannou A, Watts NB, Kendler DL, et al. Diagnosis and management of vertebral fractures in elderly adults. Am J Med 2002;113(3):220–8.

32. Lenchik L, Rogers LF, Delmas PD, et al. Diagnosis of osteoporotic vertebral fractures: importance of recognition and description by radiologists. Am J Roentgenol 2004;183(4):949–58.

33. Reddy T, McLaughlin PD, Mallinson PI, et al. Detection of occult, undisplaced hip fractures with a dual-energy CT algorithm targeted to detection of bone marrow edema. Emerg Radiol 2015; 22(1):25–9.

34. Coupal TM, Mallinson PI, McLaughlin P, et al. Peering through the glare: using dual-energy CT to overcome the problem of metal artefacts in bone radiology. Skeletal Radiol 2014;43(5):567–75.

35. Pessis E, Campagna R, Sverzut J-M, et al. Virtual monochromatic spectral imaging with fast kilovoltage switching: reduction of metal artifacts at CT. RadioGraphics 2013;33(2):573–83.

36. Wang Y, Qian B, Li B, et al. Metal artifacts reduction using monochromatic images from spectral CT: Evaluation of pedicle screws in patients with scoliosis. Eur J Radiol 2013;82(8):e360–6.

37. Lee YH, Park KK, Song H-T, et al. Metal artefact reduction in gemstone spectral imaging dual-energy CT with and without metal artefact reduction software. Eur Radiol 2012;22(6):1331–40.

38. Bamberg F, Dierks A, Nikolaou K, et al. Metal artifact reduction by dual energy computed tomography using monoenergetic extrapolation. Eur Radiol 2011; 21(7):1424–9.

39. Guggenberger R, Winklhofer S, Osterhoff G, et al. Metallic artefact reduction with monoenergetic dual-energy CT: systematic ex vivo evaluation of posterior spinal fusion implants from various vendors and different spine levels. Eur Radiol 2012; 22(11):2357–64.

40. Stolzmann P, Winklhofer S, Schwendener N, et al. Monoenergetic computed tomography reconstructions reduce beam hardening artifacts from dental restorations. Forensic Sci Med Pathol 2013;9(3): 327–32.

41. Lewis M, Reid K, Toms AP. Reducing the effects of metal artefact using high keV monoenergetic reconstruction of dual energy CT (DECT) in hip replacements. Skeletal Radiol 2013;42(2):275–82.

42. Meinel FG, Bischoff B, Zhang Q, et al. Metal artifact reduction by dual-energy computed tomography using energetic extrapolation: a systematically optimized protocol. Invest Radiol 2012;47(7):406–14.

43. Neuhaus V, Große Hokamp N, Abdullayev N, et al. Metal artifact reduction by dual-layer computed tomography using virtual monoenergetic images. Eur J Radiol 2017;93:143–8.

44. Naraghi AM, White LM. Imaging of athletic injuries of knee ligaments and menisci: sports imaging series. Radiology 2016;281(1):23–40.

45. Sunagawa T, Ishida O, Ishiburo M, et al. Three-dimensional computed tomography imaging: its applicability in the evaluation of extensor tendons in the hand and wrist. J Comput Assist Tomogr 2005;29(1):94–8.

46. Mallinson PI, Coupal TM, McLaughlin PD, et al. Dual-energy CT for the musculoskeletal system. Radiology 2016;281(3):690–707.

47. Johnson TRC, Krauß B, Sedlmair M, et al. Material differentiation by dual energy CT: initial experience. Eur Radiol 2007;17(6):1510–7.

48. Sun C, Miao F, Wang X, et al. An initial qualitative study of dual-energy CT in the knee ligaments. Surg Radiol Anat 2008;30(5):443–7.

49. Deng K, Sun C, Liu C, et al. Initial experience with visualizing hand and foot tendons by dual-energy computed tomography. Clin Imaging 2009;33(5): 384–9.

50. Fickert S, Niks M, Dinter DJ, et al. Assessment of the diagnostic value of dual-energy CT and MRI in the detection of iatrogenically induced injuries of anterior cruciate ligament in a porcine model. Skeletal Radiol 2013;42(3):411–7.

51. Peltola EK, Koskinen SK. Dual-energy computed tomography of cruciate ligament injuries in acute knee trauma. Skeletal Radiol 2015;44(9):1295–301.

52. Glazebrook KN, Brewerton LJ, Leng S, et al. Case–control study to estimate the performance of dual-energy computed tomography for anterior cruciate ligament tears in patients with history of knee trauma. Skeletal Radiol 2014;43(3):297–305.

53. Chai JW, Choi J-A, Choi J-Y, et al. Visualization of joint and bone using dual-energy CT arthrography with contrast subtraction: in vitro feasibility study using porcine joints. Skeletal Radiol 2014;43(5):673–8.

54. An C, Chun Y-M, Kim S, et al. Dual-energy computed tomography arthrography of the shoulder joint using virtual monochromatic spectral imaging: optimal dose of contrast agent and monochromatic energy level. Korean J Radiol 2014;15(6):746.

55. Subhas N, Freire M, Primak AN, et al. CT arthrography: in vitro evaluation of single and dual energy for optimization of technique. Skeletal Radiol 2010; 39(10):1025–31.

56. Murray N, Le M, Ebrahimzadeh O, et al. Imaging the spine with dual-energy CT. Curr Radiol Rep 2017; 5(9):1–12.

57. Kraus M, Weiss J, Selo N, et al. Spinal dual-energy computed tomography: improved visualisation of spinal tumorous growth with a noise-optimised advanced monoenergetic post-processing algorithm. Neuroradiology 2016;58(11):1093–102.

58. Zheng S, Dong Y, Miao Y, et al. Differentiation of osteolytic metastases and Schmorl's nodes in cancer patients using dual-energy CT: advantage of spectral CT imaging. Eur J Radiol 2014;83(7):1216–21.

59. Dong Y, Zheng S, Machida H, et al. Differential diagnosis of osteoblastic metastases from bone islands in patients with lung cancer by single-source dual-energy CT: advantages of spectral CT imaging. Eur J Radiol 2015;84(5):901–7.

60. Thomas C, Schabel C, Krauss B, et al. Dual-energy CT: virtual calcium subtraction for assessment of bone marrow involvement of the spine in multiple myeloma. Am J Roentgenol 2015;204(3):W324–31.

61. Wichmann JL, Booz C, Wesarg S, et al. Quantitative dual-energy CT for phantomless evaluation of cancellous bone mineral density of the vertebral pedicle: correlation with pedicle screw pull-out strength. Eur Radiol 2015;25(6):1714–20.

62. Mussmann B, Overgaard S, Torfing T, et al. Intra- and inter-observer agreement and reliability of bone mineral density measurements around acetabular cup: a porcine ex-vivo study using single- and dual-energy computed tomography. Acta Radiol Open 2017;6(7). 205846011771974.

63. Burge R, Dawson-Hughes B, Solomon DH, et al. Incidence and economic burden of osteoporosis-related fractures in the United States, 2005-2025. J Bone Miner Res 2007;22(3):465–75.

64. Chun KJ. Bone densitometry. Semin Nucl Med 2011; 41(3):220–8.

65. Antonacci MD, Hanson DS, Heggeness MH. Pitfalls in the measurement of bone mineral density by dual energy X-ray absorptiometry. Spine 1996; 21(1):87–90.

66. Bolotin HH, Sievänen H. Inaccuracies inherent in dual-energy X-ray absorptiometry in vivo bone mineral density can seriously mislead diagnostic/prognostic interpretations of patient-specific bone fragility. J Bone Miner Res 2001;16(5):799–805.

67. Bolotin HH. DXA in vivo BMD methodology: an erroneous and misleading research and clinical gauge of bone mineral status, bone fragility, and bone remodelling. Bone 2007;41(1):138–54.

68. Engelke K, Adams JE, Armbrecht G, et al. Clinical use of quantitative computed tomography and peripheral quantitative computed tomography in the management of osteoporosis in adults: the 2007 ISCD official positions. J Clin Densitom 2008;11(1): 123–62.

69. Damilakis J, Adams JE, Guglielmi G, et al. Radiation exposure in X-ray-based imaging techniques used in osteoporosis. Eur Radiol 2010;20(11):2707–14.

70. Wait JMS, Cody D, Jones AK, et al. Performance evaluation of material decomposition with rapid-kilovoltage-switching dual-energy CT and implications for assessing bone mineral density. Am J Roentgenol 2015;204(6):1234–41.

71. De Cecco CN, Schoepf UJ, Steinbach L, et al. White paper of the society of computed body tomography and magnetic resonance on dual-energy CT, part 3: vascular, cardiac, pulmonary, and musculoskeletal applications. J Comput Assist Tomogr 2017;41(1): 1–7.

72. Wichmann JL, Booz C, Wesarg S, et al. Dual-Energy CT–based phantomless in vivo three-dimensional bone mineral density assessment of the lumbar spine. Radiology 2014;271(3):778–84.

Dual-Energy Computed Tomography

Dose Reduction, Series Reduction, and Contrast Load Reduction in Dual-Energy Computed Tomography

Anushri Parakh, MD[a], Francesco Macri, MD, PhD[a,b], Dushyant Sahani, MD[a],*

KEYWORDS

- Dual-energy CT • Spectral CT • Radiation dose • Contrast media • Iodine • Virtual unenhanced
- Material density • Split-bolus

KEY POINTS

- Dual energy computed tomography entails balancing of radiation dose and image quality without affecting spectral separation for the clinical context being assessed.
- Existing dual energy computed tomography platforms meet diagnostic and radiation dose expectation as compared with single energy computed tomography protocols.
- Low energy virtual monochromatic (40–60 keV) images enable reduction in iodine dose while providing good contrast-to-noise ratio and image quality.
- Dual energy computed tomography can also decrease radiation and/or iodine contrast dose by decreasing the number of unequivocal scans that warrant follow-up and number of acquisitions in multiphasic examinations.

INTRODUCTION

Patient safety is paramount when adopting any new technology into clinical care. Despite the recognized clinical benefits of dual energy computed tomography (DECT), wide adoption of DECT was limited initially owing to workflow constraints and reports of higher radiation dose. Understanding the technology and its potential is key. Refinements in DECT technology, image reconstruction and material separation algorithms over the past decade has given the opportunity to optimize DECT and create double-low (radiation and contrast) protocols in accordance with basic principle of as low as reasonable achievable for good clinical practice. The ability to generate material density images (virtual unenhanced [VUE] or water images) also decreases the dose by reducing the number of true acquisitions performed in multiphasic examinations. Another indirect effect on dose reduction is the ability to reduce the absolute amount of contrast media owing to the generation of low-energy virtual monochromatic images. In addition to its

Disclosure Statement: No relevant disclosures (A. Parakh, F. Macri); Royalties from Elsevier, Research Grant from GE Healthcare and Bayer. Consultant for Allena (D. Sahani).

[a] Department of Radiology, Abdominal Imaging Division, Massachusetts General Hospital, White 270, 55 Fruit Street, Boston, MA 02114, USA; [b] Department of Radiology, University Hospital of Nimes, Place di Pr Debre, Nimes 30029, France
* Corresponding author.
E-mail address: dsahani@partners.org

Radiol Clin N Am 56 (2018) 601–624
https://doi.org/10.1016/j.rcl.2018.03.002

diagnostic and functional capability, this flexibility of DECT to reduce radiation dose, series, and contrast gives it a unique advantage over single energy CT (SECT).

We aim to provide an overview of existing evidence, and suggestions for protocols, on DECT in the perspective of improving patient care while minimizing overall exposure to ionizing radiation and iodinated contrast media.

DOSE REDUCTION

Keeping other parameters constant, the relationship between tube voltage and radiation dose is exponential, that is, a change from 120 to 140 kVp increases the radiation dose by 30% to 40%, whereas a shift from 120 to 100 or 80 kVp decreases it by 38% to 67%.[1] When DECT was first commercially available, an initial study by Ho and colleagues[2] suggested that radiation doses from DECT (80/140 kVp) were up to 3 times higher than SECT performed at 140 kVp. Such reports coupled with connotation of the word dual in the name coincided with the surging interest in medical and lay community about the potential long-term risks from ionizing radiation in medical imaging.[3] This limited early widespread clinical adoption of DECT. As a result, although truly convincing deleterious effects of cancer secondary to radiation from diagnostic imaging are debatable, considerable efforts to reduce radiation doses for all relevant modalities are being made by different stakeholders in radiology.[4] Since the initial investigations, there have been considerable refinements in hardware, software, and image reconstruction techniques for DECT to mitigate radiation dose. Furthermore, much of the initial literature did not normalize for image noise or perform image quality analysis.

Unlike SECT, in which modulating tube current is a significant factor for reducing radiation dose, optimizing radiation dose in DECT depends largely on the platform. An overview of these efforts on commercial DECT scanners is provided in **Table 1**.

Rapid kVp Switching Dual Energy Computed Tomography

This platform is limited by fixed tube current. The mA is contained by allocating a relatively longer time for 80 kVp acquisition than for 140 kVp.[5] The radiation dose is, therefore, curbed by using an appropriate gemstone spectral imaging preset that is chosen according to clinical indication and body habitus. This preset is dictated by varying combinations of tube current and pitch. Accordingly, the lowest limit of radiation dose achievable on rapid kVp switching DECT (rsDECT) is a volumetric CT dose index of 5 mGy.

Dual Source Dual Energy Computed Tomography

Tube current can be modulated in this platform, just like for SECT. There is no lower limit for

---

Table 1
Methods used by a few commercially available DECT scanners to curb radiation dose

DECT Basis	Source-Based			Detector-Based
DECT Technique	**Rapid kV Switching**	**Dual-Source**	**Twin Beam**	**Dual Layer**
Additional filtration at the x-ray tube output	None	Second- and third-generation scanners are equipped with different thickness of tin (Sn) filter at higher kVp tube	Equal halves of gold (Au) and Tin (Sn) filters at the single x-ray tube output	None
Percent low kVp state during a scan	65% scan time – 80 kVp 35% scan time – 140 kVp	Equal duration of low and high kVp states	Not applicable (single 120 kVp applied)	Not applicable (single 120 or 140 kVp applied)
Automatic tube current modulation	Not available	Available	Available	Available
Iterative reconstruction	Available	Available	Available	Available

Abbreviation: DECT, dual energy computed tomography.

radiation dose on this platform. Additionally, it uses differential filtration at the higher tube output to harden the high kVp beam by absorbing low-energy photons. Primak and colleagues[6] showed that using additional filtration in dual source DECT (dsDECT) improved material discrimination without increasing radiation dose as compared with SECT, and allows for using a higher low kVp (100 instead of 80) to increase the photon flux in larger patients with little effect on spectral overlap. Owing to the advancements in third-generation dsDECT, radiation doses incurred by the third-generation dsDECT are lower than previous generations.

The topic of radiation dose is less relevant in twin beam DECT and dual layer DECT (dlDECT) platforms when compared with 120-kVp SECT. However, investigations are needed to compare them with doses entailed by low kVp SECT scans.

Twin-Beam Dual Energy Computed Tomography

Dual filtration by gold and tin is present at the tube output that splits the x-ray beam to provide spectral information while absorbing the low-energy photons that contribute little to image formation and more toward radiation. Lower radiation doses have been observed with DECT as compared with SECT by 17% (size-specific dose estimate 9.7 mGy vs 11.7 mGy).[6-8]

Dual Layer Dual Energy Computed Tomography

This platform uses 120 or 140 kVp in conjunction with tube current modulation, it has an interlayer filter between the 2 scintillator detector layers that attenuates less than 3% of the intensity reaching the detector. Although this thin layer improves the spectral differentiation it also reduces dose efficiency. Very recently, dlDECT has become available for clinical use, and early studies assessing this technique show no significant difference from conventional SECT.[7,9]

Since the initial report by Ho and colleagues,[2] there have been growing number of reports[9-11] from phantom and patient studies in different body areas validating that scans from different DECT platforms can be performed with an acceptable radiation dose for routine clinical use with equivalent diagnostic performance.

Although few studies neglect to perform imperative image quality assessments and do not account for patient size by assessing size-specific dose estimate, many show radiation doses (volumetric CT dose index; CTDIvol) below the

suggested published reference levels and 75th percentile values by the American College of Radiology (ACR) and the ACR Dose Index Registry (Semi-Annual report 2016), respectively (**Table 2**).[12]

Moreover, most DECT protocols are also either comparable to the achievable 50th percentile ACR-Dose Index Registry volumetric CT dose index doses (abdomen, 13 mGy), or are significantly lower (pulmonary angiography, 12 mGy; head, 54 mGy; neck, 16).

Protocols for SECT are becoming more sophisticated with increasingly common use of reduced dose protocols, tube current modulation, automatic kVp selection, adaptive dose shielding, iterative reconstruction, and split-bolus techniques. Correspondingly, the dose efficiency for DECT scans is successfully evolving by using similar techniques, with comparable image noise (**Table 3**).

Another approach to reduce radiation burden is by performing targeted DECT scan in the area of interest. For instance, when evaluating for urolithiasis, where a low-dose protocol is advocated, targeted DECT acquisition in the region of the stone can be performed after a low-dose SECT acquisition.

Scanners often come with vendor recommended protocols. Just as preset protocols are optimized for SECT, the preloaded DECT protocols tend to deliver a higher radiation dose and should be calibrated before implementation. Up to 41% reduction in radiation doses can be achieved upon refining manufacturer recommended protocols, without affecting image quality or quantitative accuracy.[33]

In general, with the currently available high-end scanners, radiation doses from DECT are lower or no more than 10% to 15% higher than SECT. For scans that have a marginally higher dose penalty, the benefits of additional image reconstructions by DECT may offset these radiation dose concerns. The obvious advantages of such reconstructions that increase the diagnostic value of DECT include reduction of metal artifacts, stone composition analysis, automatic bone removal for angiographies, pulmonary perfusion, improved contrast-to-noise ratios by virtual monochromatic images, and the generation of material density iodine maps.

This postprocessing flexibility also allows for an additional reduction in DECT doses (**Fig. 1**). The improved contrast-to-noise ratio on low-energy monochromatic images and improved conspicuity on material density iodine images, can increase reader confidence and reduce the number of indeterminate interpretations (**Fig. 2**),[34] thus,

Table 2
Overview of literature show comparable radiation doses between DECT and SECT (not including reduction owing to lesser number of acquisitions)

Study, Year	n	DECT Technique	DECT kVp	Mean DECT CTDI$_{vol}$	SECT kVp	Mean SECT CTDI$_{vol}$	DECT vs SECT (%)[a]
Abdomen-pelvis (ACR-DIR 75th percentile CTDI$_{vol}$ 19 mGy)							
Shuman et al,[13] 2014	72	rsDECT	80/140	12.8	120	14.2	-9
Wichmann et al,[14] 2017	200	dsDECT; second generation	80/Sn140	14.3	120	12.9	10
	200	dsDECT; third generation	90/Sn150	7.8	100	9.2	-15
Ascenti et al,[15] 2012	70	dsDECT; first generation	80/140	13.9	120	11	2.9
Pulmonary angiography (ACR-DIR 75th percentile CTDI$_{vol}$ 16 mGy)							
Bauer et al,[16] 2011	120	dsDECT; first generation	80/140	9.2	120	8.5	8
	120	dsDECT; second generation	80/Sn140	6.2	120	8.5	-27
	120	dsDECT; second generation	100/Sn140	8.7	120	8.5	2
De Zordo et al,[17] 2012	150	dsDECT; second generation	100/Sn140	7.7	120	9.55	-18
					100	5.97	28
Petritsch et al,[18] 2017	180	dsDECT; third generation	90/Sn150	4.3	120	7.63	-43
					100	6.78	-35
Neck (ACR-DIR 75th percentile CTDI$_{vol}$ 20 mGy)							
Tawfik et al,[19] 2011	64	dsDECT; second generation	80/Sn140	10.9	120	12.4	-11
Paul et al,[20] 2013	180	dsDECT; second generation	80/Sn140	10.6	120	12.5	-15
Head (ACR-DIR 75th percentile CTDI$_{vol}$ 61 mGy)							
Kamiya et al,[21] 2013[b]	15	rsDECT	80/140	70	120	78.9	-11
Hwang et al,[22] 2016[b]	44	rsDECT	80/140	28-40	120	44-45	-11 to -36
Scholtz et al,[23] 2017[c]	122	dsDECT; third generation	80/Sn150	41	120	39.5	3

Abbreviations: ACR-DIR, American College of Radiology Dose Index Registry; CTDI$_{vol}$, volumetric computed tomography dose index; DECT, dual energy computed tomography; dsDECT, dual-source dual energy computed tomography; rsDECT, rapid kVp switching dual energy computed tomography; SECT, single energy computed tomography.
[a] (DECT-SECT)/SECT.
[b] Both performed scans on the same scanner model; however (besides differences in a rotation time and tube current) iterative reconstruction was used for the study by Hwang and colleagues not Kamiya and colleagues.
[c] Tabulated doses for Scholtz and colleagues are without automatic tube current modulation for DECT and SECT. They showed that tube current modulation reduced the doses for both DECT (29.9 mGy) and SECT (32.2 mGy).

Table 3
DECT in era of current advanced dose-efficient SECT scan techniques

Reduced dose adult protocols	• For conditions such as suspected urinary stone disease, where low-dose SECT protocols are validated, radiation doses from dsDECT in average-sized patients have been shown to be comparable to low-dose SECT[24] and intravenous pyelography[25] with minimal effect on image quality and advantage of assessing stone composition. • Using a tube current of 375 mA in rsDECT for aortoiliofemoral evaluation in average sized patients incurs reduction in radiation dose while maintaining diagnostic accuracy.[26]
Reduced dose pediatric protocols	• DECT in pediatric body CT had comparable or lower radiation doses than SECT, with maintained contrast-to-noise ratios.[8] For head DECT, the dose can be neutral to SECT doses.[27] However, when maintaining similar image quality parameters, chest DECT protocols in small children may be 11%–20% higher than SECT.
Automatic tube current modulation	• Using this technique on third-generation dsDECT resulted in a reduction of radiation dose by 24% and 26% on SECT and DECT protocols, respectively.[23]
kVp optimized protocols	• A phantom study simulating an average-sized patient showed the lowest image noise for DECT as compared with $CTDI_{vol}$-matched 100 and 120k Vp SECT protocols indicating feasibility for dose-neutral DECT to conventional and low kVp protocols.[28] • Recently, Uhrig and colleagues[29] demonstrated the feasibility of performing DECT examinations with comparable contrast-to-noise ratios and no radiation dose penalty in a large series of oncologic patients, even when using SECT with automated tube voltage selection techniques that are adapted to take into account patient habitus for scan acquisition. • With doses set to target 100kVp SECT, rsDECT with iterative reconstruction achieved doses comparable with 100 kVp SECT with iterative reconstruction.[29] Although the signal-to-noise and contrast-to-noise ratios were not significantly different, they were slightly superior for rsDECT.
IR	• With advent of IR, diagnostic quality pulmonary angiographies can be performed with rsDECT, even at a dose optimized to 100k Vp SECT.[30] • Newer generation of IR and detector configuration on third-generation dsDECT (90/150 kVp) shown to be more dose-efficient than 100 kVp SECT with similar configuration and older IR on second-generation dsDECT (80/140 kVp) or 120 kVp SECT.[14] • $CTDI_{vol}$ for head scanned on rsDECT with IR was lower than a prior study with rsDECT without IR by 30–42 mGy.[22] • IR significantly improves image quality over filtered back projection, and therefore has the potential to decrease radiation exposure.[31]
Split-bolus technique	This technique increases dose efficiency by decreasing the number of scans performed in a multiphasic examination and is commonplace in various SECT protocols. For example, a conventional triple-phase SECT urography can be reduced to 2 acquisitions by using a split bolus technique with SECT. DECT improves this capability, by potentially reducing it to a single-phase split bolus acquisition.[32]

Abbreviations: $CTDI_{vol}$, volumetric computed tomography dose index; DECT, dual energy computed tomography; dsDECT, dual-source dual energy computed tomography; IR, iterative reconstruction; rsDECT, rapid kVp switching dual energy computed tomography.

decreasing the need for unwarranted follow-up examinations and additional radiation exposure, especially for incidentalomas.[35–38] DECT can also decrease the number of series that are truly acquired in a multiphasic examination, thus, reducing the total radiation dose per examination. For example, eliminating the acquisition of a true unenhanced phase (TUE) can reduce radiation dose by almost up to 50%.[39]

As a result, radiation exposure can be additionally reduced by DECT for carefully selected applications, and this concept of series reduction as a means of dose reduction is also discussed.

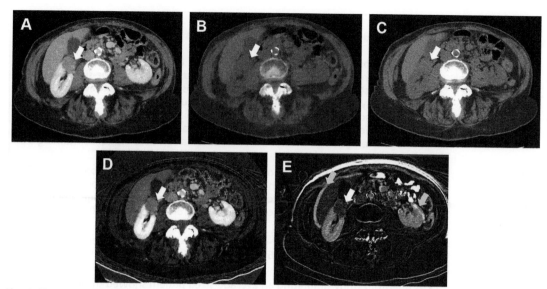

Fig. 1. Postprocessing flexibility of dual energy computed tomography demonstrated on rapid kVp switching DECT for a renal lesion. Virtual monochromatic image at 70 keV from DECT acquisition in nephrographic phase (*A*) reveals a hyperattenuating lesion (*white arrow*) arising from the anteromedial aspect of the right kidney. Virtual unenhanced reconstruction from DECT (*B*) and true unenhanced (*C*) image at 120 kVp reveal precontrast hypoattenuation within the lesion ruling out a hemorrhagic cyst and indicating a solid lesion. Material density iodine (*D*) reconstruction from DECT nulls the attenuation of background soft tissue and demonstrates the enhancement within the lesion with increased conspicuity. Although less conspicuous than a material density iodine image, a subtraction image (*E*) also reveals the degree of enhancement within the lesion. However, subtraction images are prone to misregistration artifacts, as indicated by the yellow arrows around the liver and left kidney. Radiation dose parameters: True unenhanced single-energy CT (120 kVp) – volumetric CT dose index = 14.05 mGy; dose–length product = 220.52 mGycm. Contrast-enhanced DECT (80/140 kVp)—volumetric CT dose index = 13.33 mGy; dose–length product = 361.26 mGycm.

Radiation dose is, thus, a moving target with newer limits being attained with technological advancements. In summary (**Box 1**), although multiple studies demonstrate the feasibility of performing DECT at doses within an acceptable range of SECT, various factors need to be considered while performing such comparisons and creating protocols which have doses that are as low as reasonably achievable. In this context, these factors include taking into account potential variations in doses between different generations of DECT platforms and requires careful balancing of radiation dose with image quality, without affecting spectral separation for the clinical indication. Furthermore, DECT can still not match ultralow-dose or submillisievert CT and is not recommended for screening.

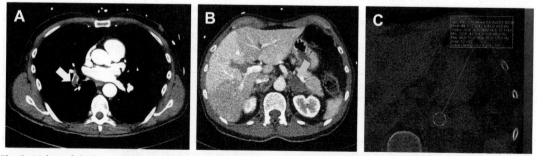

Fig. 2. Value of dual energy computed tomography (DECT) for incidentaloma. twin beam DECT (AuSn120 kVp) in a 64-year-old man with multiple thrombotic events (*A*) revealed thrombus within the segmental branches of the pulmonary artery (*white arrow*). (*B*) A hypoenhancing lesion (*yellow arrow*) was detected in the left adrenal gland which on postprocessed material density iodine overlay image (*C*) revealed an attenuation of 44 Hounsfield units on virtual unenhanced image and had no iodine uptake (0.2 mg/mL iodine), indicating a lipid-poor adenoma.

a. On currently available platforms, DECT is capable of providing similar image quality with comparable radiation dose to conventional as well as dose-optimized SECT protocols.

b. DECT doses for routine protocols are below the ACR reference values and lower or not more than 10% to 15% higher than SECT.

c. Additional image reconstructions from DECT allows for detailed problem solving, which is not possible with SECT. This decreases equivocal examinations that may need a subsequent follow-up examination involving radiation.

d. Postprocessing flexibility of DECT allows for a reduction in the number of series performed in a multiphasic scan, this has potential to further reduce the total radiation dose for an examination.

e. Task-based image quality assessment needs to be performed while evaluating radiation dose for DECT.

Abbreviations: ACR, American College of Radiology; DECT, dual energy computed tomography; SECT, single energy computed tomography.

SERIES REDUCTION

As mentioned, the ability to generate a multitude of images from a single DECT acquisition allows for reducing the number of acquisitions performed in a multiphasic examination. This unique ability provides an additional avenue for substantially minimizing radiation doses in DECT. Reduction of series can be performed in 1 of 3 ways, eliminating acquisition of a phase, combining 2 or more phases in a contrast-enhanced examination, or a combination of the two.

Eliminating an Acquisition

On VUE images, DECT suppresses the iodine distribution from a postcontrast scan. VUE, therefore, has the potential to simulate and eliminate the need for acquiring a TUE. When DECT was first commercially available for clinical use, diagnostic accuracy of VUE was one of the first evaluations performed for a DECT application. This prospective study showed the feasibility to reliably detect urinary stones on VUE images generated from nephrographic phase and suggested that this reconstruction can be used to replace TUE.[40] Since then, various studies have demonstrated that omitting TUE can significantly cut down

radiation dose by varying percentages (**Table 4**). In source-based DECT scans, which use 2 tube potentials, the elimination of 1 phase does not simply decrease the dose by one-third or one-half in triple- and dual-phase acquisitions, like it potentially would for dlDECT, that is by design performed at a single tube potential.[41]

The split-bolus technique is used in CT urography for synchronous visualization of nephrographic and excretory phases thereby reducing radiation dose. VUE further potentiates this by omitting the need for TUE and convert a 3-phase or 4-phase protocol to a biphasic or monophasic protocol.[32,48,54] However, a notable limitation is decreased sensitivity for detecting small stones on VUE. On CT angiography, Javor and colleagues[55] demonstrated a 42% reduction in radiation dose by replacing a biphasic (arterial and venous) protocol with a single split-bolus acquisition and VUE, while maintaining the diagnostic accuracy for endoleak detection and comparable image quality.

Cognizance of strengths and weaknesses of VUE is necessary before implementation. VUE can be postprocessed using all DECT techniques. Postprocessing algorithms used to generate VUE fundamentally vary across all DECT platforms, that is, 3 material decomposition on dsDECT and twin beam DECT, and 2 material or multimaterial decomposition on rsDECT. Most of the early work that assessed the accuracy of VUE have been performed on dsDECT. VUE derived from the rsDECT did not yield attenuation values (Hounsfield units [HU]) until recent refinements in multimaterial decomposition algorithms.[53] This makes generalization and application of results obtained with 1 technique onto another challenging.

Hounsfield unit on virtual unenhanced image

Overestimation or underestimation of VUE-derived HU (HU_{VUE}) may impact imaging diagnosis of certain conditions that are based on quantitative cutoff values such as adrenal adenoma, renal lesion enhancement, and hepatic steatosis. Before implementing a protocol-wide universal replacement of TUE, one must be aware of the image quality and variability between HU_{VUE} and TUE-derived HU (HU_{TUE}), the effect of phase of acquisition (arterial or venous), iodine delivery rates, and body habitus on iodine suppression in VUE.

Variability of Hounsfield unit Intrapatient analysis assessing the agreement between HU_{TUE} and HU_{VUE} report mixed results. A few studies show an overestimation of overall HU_{VUE} indicating

Table 4
Reported dose savings on eliminating 120 kVp TUE from multiphasic abdominopelvic DECT

Study, Year	Indication	DECT Platform	DECT kVp	Dose Saving (%)	Phases Acquired	Phase Suggested for Elimination
Chandarana et al,[42] 2008	Endoleak detection	dsDECT; first generation	80/140	60	TUE, arterial and delayed[a]	TUE and arterial
Stolzmann et al,[43] 2008	Endoleak detection	dsDECT; first generation	80/140	41-61[b]	TUE, arterial and delayed[a]	TUE and arterial
Graser et al,[44] 2009	Renal mass	dsDECT; first generation	80/140	35	TUE, nephrographic[a] and delayed	TUE
Graser et al,[39] 2010	Renal Mass	dsDECT; first & second generation	80/140 100/Sn140	49	TUE and nephrographic[a]	TUE
Zhang et al,[45] 2010	Liver mass	dsDECT; first generation	80/140	33	TUE, arterial[a] and venous[a]	TUE
De Cecco et al,[46] 2010	Liver mass	dsDECT; first generation	80/140	30	TUE, arterial and venous[a]	TUE
Mileto et al,[47] 2012	Pancreas	dsDECT; first generation	80/140	26	TUE, pancreatic parenchymal[a] and venous	TUE
Takeuchi et al,[48] 2012	Urography	dsDECT; first generation	80/140	52	TUE and combined nephrographic/delayed[a]	TUE
De Cecco et al,[49] 2013	Liver mass	dsDECT; second generation	80/Sn140	21	TUE, arterial[a] and venous[a]	TUE
Sun et al,[50] 2013	GI bleed	dsDECT; second generation	100/Sn140	30	TUE (from prior study), arterial and venous[a]	TUE
Chai et al,[51] 2016	Gastric mass	rsDECT	80/140	30	TUE, arterial[a] and venous[a]	TUE
De Cecco et al,[52] 2016	Liver mass	dsDECT; third generation	100/Sn150	32	TUE, arterial[a] and venous[a]	TUE
Li et al,[53] 2017	Liver mass	rsDECT	80/140	25	TUE, arterial, venous, delayed[a]	TUE

Abbreviations: DECT, dual energy computed tomography; dsDECT, dual-source dual energy computed tomography; GI, gastrointestinal; rsDECT, rapid kVp switching dual energy computed tomography; TUE, true unenhanced phase.
[a] Represents phase acquired in dual energy.
[b] Stolzmann and colleagues showed a 41% reduction on eliminating TUE only and 61% reduction on eliminating TUE and arterial phases.

incomplete subtraction of iodine,[46,49,56–58] whereas others reported an overestimation of HU_{VUE}.[52] A recent analysis on rsDECT revealed intraindividual variations in HU_{VUE} and HU_{TUE} across all organs and vessels with negligible difference in mean attenuation (ranging from -5 to 6 HU).[58] Ananthakrishnan and colleagues[41] evaluated a recently introduced dlDECT platform and found equivalent HU for all tissues except fat with no significant variability in attenuation. Zhang and colleagues,[45] Graser and colleagues,[44] and De Cecco and colleagues[52] reported no significant difference in the attenuation from venous phase–derived HU_{VUE} of liver. In contrast, Barrett and colleagues[56] and Sahni and colleagues[59] showed a small, yet statistically significant difference in the liver attenuation. Although all 5 studies use a dsDECT technique, potential reasons for the discordant findings include differences in sample size and tube potential. An evaluation of 50 patients with twin beam DECT demonstrates a maximum of 6.7 HU between TUE and VUE.[7]

Algorithms used to generate VUE vary and are based on elements that make up an organ; the variation in organ attenuations could, therefore, also be attributed to different algorithms and target organ. It may be debated that attenuation values are not absolute with reports demonstrating intrascanner and interscanner HU variations on conventional SECT acquisition.[60] Thus, small variations in HU may be of less importance. Besides, a majority of the scans across both platforms showed variability of less than 10 to 15 HU.[61] Despite such variations, studies across all 3 platforms demonstrate a strong positive correlation of HU_{VUE} with HU_{TUE}.[56]

Effect of contrast media Li and colleagues[53] found VUE derived from contrast scans with different concentration and flow rate of contrast media show TUE-equivalent signal-to-noise and contrast-to-noise ratios. This finding indicates no significant difference of concentration or flow rate on attenuation or material suppression.

Effect of body habitus Miller and colleagues[62] found a difference in attenuation when organ and body habitus correction strategies were applied. However, decreased diagnostic accuracy or image quality of VUE and increased variability HU_{VUE} has often been observed in obese patients.[40,44,59,63] Moreover, current inherent technical limitations limit the use of DECT in patients weighing more than 260 lbs (118 kg) or with a transverse diameter of more than 38 to 46 cm.[64]

Effect of phase Variable results have been demonstrated for organ attenuation on VUE derived from arterial versus venous phases. Borhani and colleagues[58] found attenuation values based on venous phase to be a better estimate of TUE attenuation with fewer cases yielding an error of greater than 10 HU. De Cecco and colleagues[49,52] found significant difference in HU derived from arterial and venous phases for kidney, spleen, pancreas, and aorta on a second-generation dsDECT, but not on third-generation dsDECT. On both generations, there was no difference in image quality and image noise between the phases. For performance of hypovascular hepatic lesion, no difference was found in detection of hypovascular lesions less than 1 cm on both generations of dsDECT. However, higher sensitivity for lesions less than 1 cm was observed for venous phase on second-generation and arterial phase on third-generation dsDECT. In evaluating first-generation dsDECT for hypovascular and hypervascular liver lesions, Zhang and colleagues[45] found higher sensitivity and image quality for arterial phase, with no significant difference in image noise. However, more number of lesions measuring less than 1 cm were missed on arterial phase. In all 3 generations, investigations showed no significant difference in lesion attenuation on both arterial and venous phases.[45,49,52] The HU_{VUE} from venous and delayed phases for assessing washout in adrenal lesions showed no significant difference; however, delayed phase provided a better estimate of lesion attenuation as compared with TUE.[65] While assessing for renal lesions and stones on VUE postprocessed from venous and excretory phases, Sahni and colleagues[59] found no difference in image noise and organ HU_{VUE} for 2 phases, but better performance for stone detection on venous phase VUE. Most studies revealed no significant difference in image noise between VUE from different phases and, as such, the phase of preference for VUE should be governed by the clinical indication.

Image quality of virtual unenhanced images
A few quantitative analyses reveal reduced image noise in dsDECT VUE as compared with TUE owing to noise reduction algorithms,[56,66] although other studies showed higher image noise for VUE.[51,58] The noise level on VUE strongly correlates with the degree of spectral separation.[59] These images are also susceptible to a few artifacts, such as rim, beam hardening, and erroneous material subtraction.[67,68] Improved spectral separation can also reduce inhomogeneous iodine suppression and inaccurate discrimination between iodine and calcium on VUE. Current literature with existing technology suggests higher performance for TUE in assessment of calcified lesions.

Nevertheless, the qualitative image analysis scores from different studies across all platforms deem VUE as diagnostically acceptable and, despite the slight subjective preference of readers toward TUE in all studies, the overall acceptance of VUE as a substitute for TUE remains high, especially with the advent of iterative reconstruction techniques.[41,44,51,56,59]

The acceptance of VUE as a replacement for TUE has been another barrier in DECT. Such perceptible differences in image quality were also observed when iterative reconstruction techniques were first introduced. Just like the radiologist's perception of iteratively reconstructed images has improved with experience, we believe that the acceptance of VUE as a surrogate for TUE for more conditions will increase as the technology continues to evolve.[69]

Clinical feasibility of virtual unenhanced images

The feasibility of using VUE has been evaluated for different pathologies (Table 5). However, owing to aforementioned variations in HU_{VUE} of different organs, with different DECT techniques, and intrinsic short comings, VUE can serve as a surrogate for TUE only in selected clinical indications at present. A thorough review of the literature focusing on the applicability of VUE in different clinical indications is beyond the scope of this article, but a few key position papers highlighting its current status have been published. In general, VUE also been shown to have a higher performance than TUE for the detection of hypodense lesions, probably owing to the additional tin filtration and/or improved contrast owing to a lower tube potential.[6,51,52,56,67] Recent white papers by the ACR Incidental Findings Committees have validated the use of VUE for incidentally encountered adrenal and hepatic lesions.[70,71] In consensus, an expert panel on DECT across 8 institutions recently recommended the use of VUE as a surrogate for TUE; thus, changing a triple phase (TUE, arterial/parenchymal, and venous) liver and pancreatic protocol to a dual-phase protocol, with DECT acquisition performed in the arterial phase.[64,69] VUE was also suggested to replace TUE when evaluating for mesenteric ischemia or gastrointestinal bleed, with DECT being performed for both the arterial and venous phases. It cannot, at present, replace TUE for renal examinations. Figs. 3 and 4 provide examples of VUE in a few abdominal conditions.

As new DECT techniques and material decomposition algorithms are continuously being introduced, optimized and increasingly used, the use of VUE is gaining popularity and needs further validation for other clinical indications and generalization across different platforms.

Combining Two Acquisitions

The increased analytical capability of DECT helps to acquire a single phase with adequate contrast-to-noise ratio that is otherwise obtained by performing 2 phases. This method of dose reduction is further potentiated by omitting a TUE acquisition.

With a single split-bolus protocol that enabled visualization of corticomedullary, nephrographic and excretory phases, Chen and colleagues[81] demonstrated excellent enhancement of parenchyma, vessels, and the urinary tract. Iodine overlay images along with VUE (DECT interpretation) had a slightly superior performance than TUE with weighted average image (SECT interpretation) for detecting urothelial lesions. They reported a dose saving from 15.4 to 6.7 mV on replacing VUE with TUE.

Wang and colleagues[82] compared a split-bolus DECT acquisition that combined corticomedullary and nephrographic phases (including VUE) with a triphasic SECT examination (TUE, corticomedullary, and nephrographic). Their study revealed an improved lesion-to-kidney contrast ratio at 58 keV and renal vein enhancement at 67 keV than conventional corticomedullary and nephrographic phases, respectively. The DECT protocol showed an improved or equivalent performance to SECT protocol with a 28% reduced radiation dose.

Evaluation of pancreatic lesions in 163 patients with split-bolus technique DECT acquisition that combined parenchymal and venous phases showed a reduction in radiation dose by 43% with comparable to increased lesion conspicuity on 60 keV monochromatic images than individual parenchymal and venous phases.[83]

In summary (Box 2), without significantly affecting image quality, using an optimized protocol, iterative reconstruction, and eliminating TUE in DECT can significantly decrease radiation doses to levels much lower than those for SECT.

CONTRAST REDUCTION

Contrast media has been considered as the third most common cause of hospital-acquired acute kidney injury.[84] Despite recent reports that state the risk of nephropathy secondary to contrast media as debatable, good clinical practice involves administering as low a dose as diagnostically acceptable.[85] Another reason to reduce the amount of contrast is that recent studies postulate the association of iodinated contrast media and

Table 5
Details of studies evaluating VUE images as a surrogate for TUE images for lesion detection or characterization in the abdomen

Authors	Lesion Type	Sample Size	DECT Platform Generation	Phase of VUE	Statistically Significant HU$_{TUE}$ vs HU$_{VUE}$	VUE IQ Analysis		Performance
						Objective	Subjective	
Adrenal								
Ho et al,[72] 2012	Adenoma vs nonadenoma	19	dsDECT First generation (80/140)	Venous	No difference in mean HU for all lesions Mean HU$_{VUE}$ overestimation by Δ1.8 HU	No significant difference in image noise	NA	Diagnostic agreement between TUE and VUE for distinguishing benign and malignant nodules
Botsikas et al,[65] 2014	Adrenal Lesion characterization	21	dsDECT Second generation (100/Sn140)	Venous and delayed	Higher lesion HU$_{VUE}$ on venous phase (Δ12.6 HU) No difference with delayed phase HU$_{VUE}$ (Δ4.02 HU) Mean value of washout from venous phase VUE different than TUE and delayed phase VUE	NA	NA	Owing to overestimation of HU$_{VUE}$, threshold of 10 HU can be used to diagnose adrenal adenoma
Renal								
Graser et al,[44] 2009	Renal mass benign vs malignant	202	dsDECT First generation (80/140); and dsDECT Second generation (100/Sn140)	Nephrographic	NA	NA	TUE significantly better Significantly higher noise on VUE Image quality of VUE on second generation dsDECT scored better than first generation	No significant difference in accuracy of lesion characterization

(continued on next page)

Table 5
(continued)

Authors	Lesion Type	Sample Size	DECT Platform	Phase of VUE Generation	Statistically Significant HU$_{TUE}$ vs HU$_{VUE}$	VUE IQ Analysis			Performance
						Objective	Subjective		
Neville et al,[73] 2011	Renal mass benign vs malignant	139	dsDECT First generation (80/140)	Nephrographic	No difference in lesion or degree of enhancement attenuation	No difference	NA		Lesion characterization with VUE is within limits of agreement
Song et al,[74] 2011	Renal mass benign vs malignant	60	dsDECT Second generation (80/Sn140)	Corticomedullary and nephrographic	No difference in lesion attenuation Difference in liver and psoas HU on VUE from both phases Difference in aortic HU on VUE from corticomedullary phase	NA	IQ of VUE inferior to TUE IQ of corticomedullary phase better than nephrographic All images fair or better		Accurate characterization possible
Liver									
Tian et al,[75] 2015	Hepatic metastasis	40	rsDECT (80/140)	Arterial, venous and delayed	NA	Contrast-to-noise ratio for arterial phase VUE better than TUE Other phases VUE equivalent to TUE	No difference with arterial and venous derived VUE IQ for delayed phase VUE worse		No difference in metastatic detection rate across all VUE

Study	n	DECT type	Phase	HU findings	Image noise findings	IQ findings	Conclusion
Gall Bladder							
Kim et al,[76] 2012	100	dsDECT First generation (80/140)	Arterial and venous	HU of stone and stone size underestimated on VUE; HU of liver, bile and muscle significantly different	Less image noise on both VUE; Contrast-to-noise ratio best for VUE from venous phase > arterial phase > TUE	Excellent IQ in 95%–97% cases; Others were rated fair	VUE from arterial phase accepted in 89%–90% cases, (reasonable) with limited role in stones <1.7 mm or HU <78; VUE underestimate stone size
Lee et al,[77] 2016		dsDECT Second generation (80/Sn140)	Venous	HU$_{VUE}$ significantly higher for liver and muscle, and lower for bile	Contrast-to-noise ratio of cholesterol stones higher on VUE, but lower for calcium stones	VUE showed higher image noise, with acceptable images in 69%–71% cases and acceptable with restrictions in 25%	Underestimation of stone size on VUE; Visibility of cholesterol stone better on VUE; TUE better for calcium-based and small-sized stones
Pancreas							
Mileto et al,[47] 2012	51	dsDECT First generation (80/140)	Parenchymal	NA	Statistically significant lower image noise in VUE	No difference in IQ	NA
Bowel							
Chen et al,[78] 2014	103	dsDECT Second generation (80/Sn140)	Venous	No concordance but HU correlation of normal organ and tumor	No difference in image noise	No to minimal noise for both TUE and VUE; IQ score significantly better for TUE, but excellent for both	Completely acceptable to replace VUE with TUE; No deterioration of accuracy for tumor detection

(continued on next page)

Table 5
(continued)

Authors	Lesion Type	Sample Size	DECT Platform	Phase of VUE Generation	Statistically Significant HU_{TUE} vs HU_{VUE}	VUE IQ Analysis Objective	VUE IQ Analysis Subjective	Performance
Sun et al,[79] 2015	Active gastrointestinal bleed	112	dsDECT Second generation (100/Sn140)	Venous	No difference in mean HU_{VUE} of all organs	Statistically significant lower image noise and higher signal-to-noise ratio for VUE	No significant difference, but lower IQ for VUE	No difference in bleed detection when using VUE
Chai et al,[51] 2016	Gastric tumors	95	rsDECT (80/140)	Arterial	Mean HU_{VUE} of lesion and metastasis higher than HU_{TUE} (Δ2.32 and Δ1.97 HU) No difference in relative enhancement HU_{VUE} of aorta higher by mean Δ4.3HU No difference in HU of liver, muscle and lymph node	Contrast-to-noise ratio of tumor to gastric lumen higher for VUE than TUE Image noise for VUE higher than TUE	No significant difference in IQ	Comparable diagnostic accuracy for VUE and TUE
Angiography								
Stolzmann et al,[43] 2008	Endoleak detection	118	dsDECT First generation (80/140)	Delayed	NA	NA	NA	No difference in endoleak detection when using VUE
Flors et al,[80] 2013	Endoleak detection	48	dsDECT First generation (80/140)	Delayed	No difference in luminal aortic measurement	NA	NA	No difference in endoleak detection when using VUE

Abbreviations: DECT, dual energy computed tomography; dsDECT, dual-source dual energy computed tomography; HU, Hounsfield unit; HU_{TUE}, true unenhanced phase-derived Hounsfield unit; HU_{VUE}, virtual unenhanced phase-derived Hounsfield unit; IQ, image quality; NA, not applicable; rsDECT, rapid kVp switching dual energy computed tomography; TUE, true unenhanced phase; VUE, virtual unenhanced image.

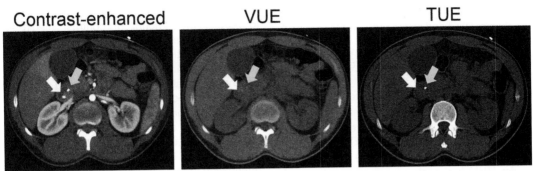

Fig. 3. Virtual unenhanced image (VUE) reconstruction from dual-source dual energy computed tomography (CT) technique in gastrointestinal hemorrhage. Weighted-average image reveals active extravasation of intravenous iodinated contrast (*white arrow*) within the duodenum on arterial phase contrast-enhanced images, which is not visualized on corresponding VUE and true unenhanced phase images, indicating active gastrointestinal hemorrhage. Note the partial subtraction of pancreatic stent (*yellow arrow*) and 'smoothened' appearance of structures in VUE. Radiation dose parameters: True unenhanced single-energy CT (110 kVp) – volumetric CT dose index = 4.89 mGy; dose–length product = 250.3 mGycm. Contrast-enhanced DECT (100/Sn 150 kVp)-volumetric CT dose index = 5.80 mGy; dose–length product = 286 mGycm.

increased radiation doses, leading to an increase in the number of double-strand DNA breaks.[86]

Optimal enhancement is influenced by scan parameters (low kVp or low keV, scan timing and delay), contrast media factors (iodine concentration, volume, injection rate, and duration), and patient factors (cardiac output, body weight). Conventionally, 120 kVp abdominal CT angiography is performed with approximately 35 to 50 g of iodine with a 3.5 to 4.0 mL/s flow rate and a 25- to 30-s injection duration to achieve a target aortic attenuation of greater than 200 HU.[87,88]

As the keV of the virtual monochromatic dataset is decreased and approaches the k-edge of iodine, it results in viewing a larger proportion of photons that interact with iodine (**Fig. 5**). When compared with 77 keV (mean energy of polyenergetic 120

kVp beam), the average attenuation of iodine increases by 25% at 70 keV (approximately 100 kVp) and 70% at 60 keV (approximately 80kVp).[89] DECT-generated virtual monochromatic or monoenergetic datasets with energy ranging from 40 to 70 keV can thus be exploited to reduce the amount of administered iodine dose without decreasing the contrast-to-noise ratio.

The concept of using low tube voltage in SECT examinations to achieve high contrast-to-noise ratios in vascular studies while reducing iodine (and radiation dose) has been extensively studied (**Table 6**).[90] However, lowering the kVp comes at the cost of increased image noise that requires tailoring of tube current, pitch, and/or iterative reconstruction in compensation. DECT allows the flexibility of creating low keV (high contrast

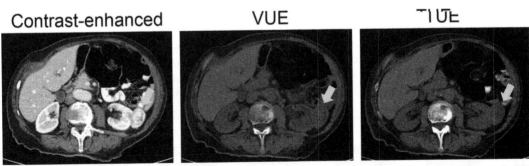

Fig. 4. Virtual unenhanced image (VUE) reconstruction from dual-layer dual energy computed tomography (CT) technique in renal cell carcinoma. A 120 kVp image demonstrates heterogeneously enhancing lesion arising from the left renal cortex (*yellow arrow*). VUE and true unenhanced phase have a comparable image quality and confirm presence of enhancement, clinching the diagnosis of renal cell carcinoma. Note the suppression of oral contrast media on VUE. Radiation dose parameters: True unenhanced single-energy CT (120 kVp) – volumetric CT dose index = 7.7 mGy; dose–length product = 271.1 mGycm. Contrast-enhanced dual energy CT (120 kVp) – volumetric CT dose index = 9.5 mGy; dose–length product = 610 mGycm.

and noise) for vascular assessment and high keV images (lower contrast and noise) for assessing soft tissue. In addition, the high keV images assist in metal artifact reduction, which could be helpful in the presence of stents and implants. Furthermore, recently introduced noise-optimized monoenergetic images possess high iodine-attenuating characteristics of a low energy dataset with the low image noise characteristics of a high-energy dataset, which allows a balance between the contrast-to-noise ratio for the evaluation of vascular and nonvascular structures. Iterative reconstruction techniques further improve the image quality of monochromatic images.[91–93]

Accumulating evidence suggests the feasibility to reduce the amount of contrast media for vascular studies while maintaining diagnostically acceptable aortic intravascular attenuation using DECT (see **Table 6**). Recent studies on a rsDECT scanner have shown that 21 to 27 g of iodine at 50 keV yielded 60% to 92% higher aortic attenuation as compared with 30 to 52 g of iodine at 120 kVp with comparable signal-to-noise and contrast-to-noise ratios.[94,95] Further reduction to 15 g at 50 keV demonstrated comparable aortic attenuation (approximately 338HU), signal-to-noise and contrast-to-noise ratios with 50 g of iodine at 120 kVp.[88] **Fig. 6** shows a CT angiogram with serially reduced iodine doses.

Reduced iodine exposure has also been evaluated for CT pulmonary angiography extensively, with a study demonstrating the feasibility of using as little as 6 g of iodine.[103] Recent studies have also evaluated using reduced iodine dose for peripheral and coronary CT angiographies.[104,105]

A reduction of concentration or volume necessitates altering injection protocols. Notably, at a constant iodine flux with a similar iodine dose, the concentration of contrast agent does not impact attenuation level.[106] A lower iodine flux can, to a certain degree, be compensated by the substantial attenuation gain achieved on low keV image reconstructions.[94] However, in general a reduced iodine dose protocol for the same injection duration requires a slower flow rate to maintain iodine flux; this is additionally beneficial in patients with poor intravenous access.[107] With current SECT protocols, an injection rate of at least 3.0 mL/s is necessary for adequate duration of optimal vascular and parenchymal enhancement.[108] Conversely, a reduced iodine dose protocol with the same injection rate requires a longer injection duration or increase in volume through appropriate dilution to achieve a uniform magnitude of vascular enhancement.[108]

Very few studies have investigated reduced iodine protocols for nonvascular examinations that require optimal low-contrast detectability. In an animal model, Chung and colleagues[109] found that, for achieving comparable contrast-to-noise

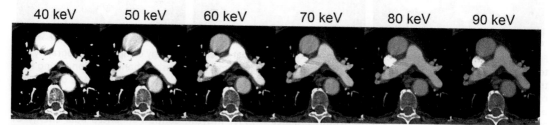

Fig. 5. Increase in iodine attenuation on decreasing the kilo electron volt in virtual monochromatic images.

Table 6
Studies assessing different iodine doses for aortic evaluation with low tube voltage and DECT

Author	Tube Voltage (kVp)	Volume (mL)	Concentration (mg I/mL)	Mean Iodine Dose (g)
Tube voltage selection technique				
Iezzi et al,[96] 2011	120	120	300	36
	80	90	400	36
Goetti et al,[97] 2012	80–140	80	300	24
Ippolito et al,[98] 2015	120	80	350	28
	100	30	350	10.5
Higashigaito et al,[99] 2016	80–110	33–68	400	13.2–27.2
Nijhof et al,[100] 2016	80	30	350	10.5
DECT technique				
Carrascosa et al,[87] 2014	120	90.3	350	31
	80/140	39.5		13.8
	80/140	28.3		9.9
	80/140	23.9		8.3
Xin et al,[101] 2015	120	91	350	32
	80/140	87	270	23
He et al,[102] 2015	120	97–138	370	36–51
	80/140	95–130	300	28–38
Agrawal et al,[94] 2016	120	80–100	370	33.3
	80/140	80–100/75	270/320	24
Shuman et al,[95] 2016	120	120–150	350	47
	80/140	81–96	270	24
Shuman et al,[88] 2017	120	100–150	350	50
	80/140	NA	270/350	15

Abbreviation: DECT, dual energy computed tomography.

ratios, hypovascular lesions can tolerate a smaller percentage of iodine dose reduction as compared with hypervascular lesions. In patients with suspected liver or pancreatic lesions, Clark and colleagues[110] demonstrated that 37% reduction in contrast media (29–70 g vs 19–46 g of iodine) on 52 keV images resulted in improved lesion to parenchyma contrast, comparable contrast-to-noise ratio and good image quality. Although early reports are promising, more studies evaluating nonangiographic reduced iodine protocols are warranted. On a recently introduced dIDECT, a potential reduction of 50% iodine at 50 keV images with comparable or better contrast-to-noise ratio has been demonstrated across scans over various body regions.[111]

120 kVp, 33 g Iodine   50 keV, 25 g Iodine   50 keV, 16 g Iodine

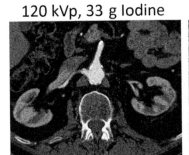 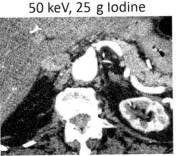 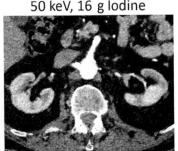

Fig. 6. Serial reduction of iodine dose in our practice. Examples of image quality and vascular enhancement during arterial phase single-energy CT acquisition performed at 120 kVp with 33 g iodine, and dual energy computed tomography with virtual monochromatic image at 50 keV with 25 and 16 g iodine.

Box 3
Highlights: DECT and contrast reduction

a. Substantial gain in attenuation of iodine on low energy (kVp or keV) images allow for reduction in intravenous and positive oral contrast media dose.

b. Compared with low kVp images with higher noise, DECT allows creation of low keV images with improved contrast and high keV images with low image noise.

c. Noise optimized virtual monoenergetic images and iterative reconstruction techniques improve image quality at lower keV images allowing for reduction in iodine dose.

d. Reduced iodine dose necessitates resetting of injection protocols (injection rate or duration) to maintain adequate iodine flux for the clinical indication.

e. Low keV (40–60) images provide a good balance of contrast-to-noise ratio and image quality with reduced iodine protocols.

Abbreviation: DECT, dual energy computed tomography.

Parallel to reducing intravenous contrast dose, low-energy scanning with automated tube voltage selection techniques and low keV images also increases the attenuation of positive oral contrast media. The gain in attenuation at these energies can lead to substantial artifacts, increase tube current demand, or impede visualization of bowel pathologies. This also provides an opportunity to change the existing protocols for positive oral contrast media and reduce

---

Table 7
Protocol used in our institution for oncologic surveillance and suspected gastrointestinal hemorrhage

Parameters	Cancer Follow-up[a] with DECT in Portovenous Phase		Mesenteric or Gastrointestinal Hemorrhage with DECT in Arterial Phase	
	rsDECT	dsDECT Second Generation	rsDECT	dsDECT Second Generation
True unenhanced	Not acquired	Not acquired	Not acquired	Not acquired
Phase acquired	Portovenous Delayed if necessary	Portovenous Delayed if necessary	Arterial, portovenous Delayed if necessary	Arterial, portovenous Delayed if necessary
kVp	80/140	80/Sn140	80/140	80/Sn140
mA	<150 lbs – 375 150–250 lbs- 630	200 with tube current modulation	<150 lbs – 600 150–250 lbs- 640	200 with tube current modulation
Rotation time	<150 lbs – 0.7 150–250 lbs- 0.5	0.5	<150 lbs – 0.6 150–250 lbs- 0.8	0.33
Pitch/speed	<150 lbs – 1.375/55 150–250 lbs- 0.984/39.37	0.95	<150 lbs – 1.375/55 150–250 lbs- 0.984/39.37	0.95
Iterative reconstruction	ASiR 50%	SAFIRE-3	ASiR 50%	SAFIRE-3
Images to PACS	Quality check, monochromatic 65 keV, material density iodine, VUE	80 kVp, 140 SnkVp, weighted average, material density iodine, VUE	Quality check, monochromatic 65 keV, material density iodine, VUE	80 kVp, 140 SnkVp, weighted average, material density iodine, VUE

Abbreviations: ASiR, adaptive statistical iterative reconstruction; DECT, dual energy computed tomography; dsDECT, dual-source dual energy computed tomography; PACS, picture archiving and communication system; rsDECT, rapid kVp switching dual energy computed tomography; SAFIRE, sinogram affirmed iterative reconstruction; VUE, virtual unenhanced image.
[a] For all cancer follow-up except bladder, pancreas, and hepatocellular.

dose for both barium and iodine by 25% to 75%.[112]

In addition to improved patient safety, reducing contrast media can also contribute as a departmental cost-savings measure.[113,114]

In summary (**Box 3**), the development and increased availability of CT technology such as iterative reconstruction and DECT have improved image quality, while opening new perspectives on creation of customized acquisition parameters that allow for a reduction in iodine exposure.

SUGGESTIONS FOR PROTOCOL DEVELOPMENT

To reiterate, the protocols for DECT need to be optimized according to the clinical question and each scan requires balancing image quality with radiation exposure and iodine dose. Depending on the platform, we recommend a few suggestions on rsDECT and second-generation dsDECT scanners for 2 weight-based abdominopelvic protocols (**Table 7**). We do not perform DECT scans in patients weighing more than 250 lbs across the DECT techniques.

SUMMARY

Radiation and iodine doses require balancing of image quality, spectral separation, and overall diagnostic performance of DECT and are moving targets. Despite the name, DECT does not entail twice the amount of radiation dose as compared with conventional SECT. Iterative reconstruction techniques have played a significant role in improving image quality and enable double dose (radiation and iodinated contrast) savings with DECT. These new techniques have, therefore, introduced the feasibility of maximizing clinical benefit by performing more sophisticated and customized protocols, which are capable of providing functional information while ensuring diagnostic efficiency and patient safety. Beside improving patient safety, reduced-phase protocols by DECT also have the possibility of improving patient throughput. It should be kept in mind, however, that generalization of results is difficult at present, owing to variations in quantitative and qualitative parameters that exist owing to differences in DECT techniques between vendors.

REFERENCES

1. McNitt-Gray MF. AAPM/RSNA physics tutorial for residents: topics in CT. Radiation dose in CT. Radiographics 2002;22(6):1541–53.
2. Ho LM, Yoshizumi TT, Hurwitz LM, et al. Dual energy versus single energy MDCT: measurement of radiation dose using adult abdominal imaging protocols. Acad Radiol 2009;16(11):1400–7.
3. Nickoloff EL, Alderson PO. Radiation exposures to patients from CT: reality, public perception, and policy. AJR Am J Roentgenol 2001;177(2):285–7.
4. Parakh A, Kortesniemi M, Schindera ST. CT radiation dose management: a comprehensive optimization process for improving patient safety. Radiology 2016;280(3):663–73.
5. Kaza RK, Platt JF, Cohan RH, et al. Dual-energy CT with single- and dual-source scanners: current applications in evaluating the genitourinary tract. Radiographics 2012;32(2):353–69.
6. Primak AN, Giraldo JC, Eusemann CD, et al. Dual-source dual-energy CT with additional tin filtration: dose and image quality evaluation in phantoms and in vivo. AJR Am J Roentgenol 2010;195(5): 1164–74.
7. Euler A, Parakh A, Falkowski AL, et al. Initial results of a single-source dual-energy computed tomography technique using a split-filter: assessment of image quality, radiation dose, and accuracy of dual-energy applications in an in vitro and in vivo study. Invest Radiol 2016;51(8):491–8.
8. Siegel MJ, Curtis WA, Ramirez-Giraldo JC. Effects of dual-energy technique on radiation exposure and image quality in pediatric body CT. AJR Am J Roentgenol 2016;207(4):826–35.
9. Hojjati M, Van Hedent S, Rassouli N, et al. Quality of routine diagnostic abdominal images generated from a novel detector-based spectral CT scanner: a technical report on a phantom and clinical study. Abdom Radiol (NY) 2017;42(11):2752–9.
10. Zhang D, Li X, Liu B. Objective characterization of GE discovery CT750 HD scanner: gemstone spectral imaging mode. Med Phys 2011;38(3):1178–88.
11. Li B, Yadava G, Hsieh J. Quantification of head and body CTDI(VOL) of dual-energy x-ray CT with fast-kVp switching. Med Phys 2011;38(5):2595–601.
12. Semiannual report-adult, Jul-Dec2016. American College of Radiology Website. 2017. Available at: https://www.acr.org/~/media/ACR/Documents/PDF/QualitySafety/NRDR/DIR/DIRSampleReport.pdf?la=en. Accessed October 9, 2017.
13. Shuman WP, Green DE, Busey JM, et al. Dual-energy liver CT: effect of monochromatic imaging on lesion detection, conspicuity, and contrast-to-noise ratio of hypervascular lesions on late arterial phase. AJR Am J Roentgenol 2014;203(3):601–6.
14. Wichmann JL, Hardie AD, Schoepf UJ, et al. Single- and dual-energy CT of the abdomen: comparison of radiation dose and image quality of 2nd and 3rd generation dual-source CT. Eur Radiol 2017; 27(2):642–50.
15. Ascenti G, Mazziotti S, Mileto A, et al. Dual-source dual-energy CT evaluation of complex cystic renal masses. AJR Am J Roentgenol 2012;199(5):1026–34.

16. Bauer RW, Kramer S, Renker M, et al. Dose and image quality at CT pulmonary angiography-comparison of first and second generation dual-energy CT and 64-slice CT. Eur Radiol 2011; 21(10):2139–47.

17. De Zordo T, von Lutterotti K, Dejaco C, et al. Comparison of image quality and radiation dose of different pulmonary CTA protocols on a 128-slice CT: high-pitch dual source CT, dual energy CT and conventional spiral CT. Eur Radiol 2012; 22(2):279–86.

18. Petritsch B, Kosmala A, Gassenmaier T, et al. Diagnosis of pulmonary artery embolism: comparison of single-source CT and 3rd generation dual-source CT using a dual-energy protocol regarding image quality and radiation dose. Rofo 2017;189(6): 527–36.

19. Tawfik AM, Kerl JM, Razek AA, et al. Image quality and radiation dose of dual-energy CT of the head and neck compared with a standard 120-kVp acquisition. AJNR Am J Neuroradiol 2011;32(11): 1994–9.

20. Paul J, Mbalisike EC, Nour-Eldin NE, et al. Dual-source 128-slice MDCT neck: radiation dose and image quality estimation of three different protocols. Eur J Radiol 2013;82(5):787–96.

21. Kamiya K, Kunimatsu A, Mori H, et al. Preliminary report on virtual monochromatic spectral imaging with fast kVp switching dual energy head CT: comparable image quality to that of 120-kVp CT without increasing the radiation dose. Jpn J Radiol 2013; 31(4):293–8.

22. Hwang WD, Mossa-Basha M, Andre JB, et al. Qualitative comparison of noncontrast head dual-energy computed tomography using rapid voltage switching technique and conventional computed tomography. J Comput Assist Tomogr 2016;40(2): 320–5.

23. Scholtz JE, Wichmann JL, Bennett DW, et al. Detecting intracranial hemorrhage using automatic tube current modulation with advanced modeled iterative reconstruction in unenhanced head single- and dual-energy dual-source CT. AJR Am J Roentgenol 2017;208(5):1089–96.

24. Jepperson MA, Cernigliaro JG, Ibrahim el-SH, et al. In vivo comparison of radiation exposure of dual-energy CT versus low-dose CT versus standard CT for imaging urinary calculi. J Endourol 2015; 29(2):141–6.

25. Thomas C, Heuschmid M, Schilling D, et al. Urinary calculi composed of uric acid, cystine, and mineral salts: differentiation with dual-energy CT at a radiation dose comparable to that of intravenous pyelography. Radiology 2010;257(2):402–9.

26. Dubourg B, Caudron J, Lestrat JP, et al. Single-source dual-energy CT angiography with reduced iodine load in patients referred for aortoiliofemoral evaluation before transcatheter aortic valve implantation: impact on image quality and radiation dose. Eur Radiol 2014;24(11):2659–68.

27. Zhu X, McCullough WP, Mecca P, et al. Dual-energy compared to single-energy CT in pediatric imaging: a phantom study for DECT clinical guidance. Pediatr Radiol 2016;46(12):1671–9.

28. Schick D, Pratap J. Radiation dose efficiency of dual-energy CT benchmarked against single-source, kilovoltage-optimized scans. Br J Radiol 2016;89(1058):20150486.

29. Uhrig M, Simons D, Kachelrieß M, et al. Advanced abdominal imaging with dual energy CT is feasible without increasing radiation dose. Cancer Imaging 2016;16(1):15.

30. Ohana M, Labani A, Jeung MY, et al. Iterative reconstruction in single source dual-energy CT pulmonary angiography: is it sufficient to achieve a radiation dose as low as state-of-the-art single-energy CTPA? Eur J Radiol 2015;84(11):2314–20.

31. Wang R, Yu W, Wu R, et al. Improved image quality in dual-energy abdominal CT: comparison of iterative reconstruction in image space and filtered back projection reconstruction. AJR Am J Roentgenol 2012;199(2):402–6.

32. Toepker M, Kuehas F, Kienzl D, et al. Dual energy computerized tomography with a split bolus-a 1-stop shop for patients with suspected urinary stones? J Urol 2014;191(3):792–7.

33. Schindera ST, Zaehringer C, D'Errico L, et al. Systematic radiation dose optimization of abdominal dual-energy CT on a second-generation dual-source CT scanner: assessment of the accuracy of iodine uptake measurement and image quality in an in vitro and in vivo investigations. Abdom Radiol (NY) 2017;42(10):2562–70.

34. Kulkarni NM, Sahani DV, Desai GS, et al. Indirect computed tomography venography of the lower extremities using single-source dual-energy computed tomography: advantage of low-kiloelectron volt monochromatic images. J Vasc Interv Radiol 2012; 23(7):879–86.

35. Mileto A, Nelson RC, Marin D, et al. Dual-energy multidetector CT for the characterization of incidental adrenal nodules: diagnostic performance of contrast-enhanced material density analysis. Radiology 2015;274(2):445–54.

36. Mileto A, Nelson RC, Samei E, et al. Impact of dual-energy multi-detector row CT with virtual monochromatic imaging on renal cyst pseudoenhancement: in vitro and in vivo study. Radiology 2014; 272(3):767–76.

37. Yamada Y, Yamada M, Sugisawa K, et al. Renal cyst pseudoenhancement: intraindividual comparison between virtual monochromatic spectral images and conventional polychromatic 120-kVp images obtained during the same CT examination

and comparisons among images reconstructed using filtered back projection, adaptive statistical iterative reconstruction, and model-based iterative reconstruction. Medicine (Baltimore) 2015;94(15): e754.

38. Slebocki K, Kraus B, Chang DH, et al. Incidental findings in abdominal dual-energy computed tomography: correlation between true noncontrast and virtual noncontrast images considering renal and liver cysts and adrenal masses. J Comput Assist Tomogr 2017;41(2):294–7.

39. Graser A, Becker CR, Staehler M, et al. Single-phase dual-energy CT allows for characterization of renal masses as benign or malignant. Invest Radiol 2010;45(7):399–405.

40. Scheffel H, Stolzmann P, Frauenfelder T, et al. Dual-energy contrast-enhanced computed tomography for the detection of urinary stone disease. Invest Radiol 2007;42(12):823–9.

41. Ananthakrishnan L, Rajiah P, Ahn R, et al. Spectral detector CT-derived virtual non-contrast images: comparison of attenuation values with unenhanced CT. Abdom Radiol (NY) 2017;42(3):702–9.

42. Chandarana H, Godoy MC, Vlahos I, et al. Abdominal aorta: evaluation with dual-source dual-energy multidetector CT after endovascular repair of aneurysms–initial observations. Radiology 2008; 249(2):692–700.

43. Stolzmann P, Frauenfelder T, Pfammatter T, et al. Endoleaks after endovascular abdominal aortic aneurysm repair: detection with dual-energy dual-source CT. Radiology 2008;249(2):682–91.

44. Graser A, Johnson TR, Hecht EM, et al. Dual-energy CT in patients suspected of having renal masses: can virtual nonenhanced images replace true nonenhanced images? Radiology 2009; 252(2):433–40.

45. Zhang LJ, Peng J, Wu SY, et al. Liver virtual nonenhanced CT with dual-source, dual-energy CT: a preliminary study. Eur Radiol 2010;20(9):2257–64.

46. De Cecco CN, Buffa V, Fedeli S, et al. Dual energy CT (DECT) of the liver: conventional versus virtual unenhanced images. Eur Radiol 2010;20(12): 2870–5.

47. Mileto A, Mazziotti S, Gaeta M, et al. Pancreatic dual-source dual-energy CT: is it time to discard unenhanced imaging? Clin Radiol 2012;67(4): 334–9.

48. Takeuchi M, Kawai T, Ito M, et al. Split-bolus CT-urography using dual-energy CT: feasibility, image quality and dose reduction. Eur J Radiol 2012; 81(11):3160–5.

49. De Cecco CN, Darnell A, Macías N, et al. Virtual unenhanced images of the abdomen with second-generation dual-source dual-energy computed tomography: image quality and liver lesion detection. Invest Radiol 2013;48(1):1–9.

50. Sun H, Xue HD, Wang YN, et al. Dual-source dual-energy computed tomography angiography for active gastrointestinal bleeding: a preliminary study. Clin Radiol 2013;68(2):139–47.

51. Chai Y, Xing J, Gao J, et al. Feasibility of virtual nonenhanced images derived from single-source fast kVp-switching dual-energy CT in evaluating gastric tumors. Eur J Radiol 2016;85(2):366–72.

52. De Cecco CN, Muscogiuri G, Schoepf UJ, et al. Virtual unenhanced imaging of the liver with third-generation dual-source dual-energy CT and advanced modeled iterative reconstruction. Eur J Radiol 2016;85(7):1257–64.

53. Li Y, Jackson A, Li X, et al. Comparison of virtual unenhanced CT images of the abdomen under different iodine flow rates. Abdom Radiol (NY) 2017;42(1):312–21.

54. Karlo CA, Gnannt R, Winklehner A, et al. Split-bolus dual-energy CT urography: protocol optimization and diagnostic performance for the detection of urinary stones. Abdom Imaging 2013;38(5): 1136–43.

55. Javor D, Wressnegger A, Unterhumer S, et al. Endoleak detection using single-acquisition split-bolus dual-energy computer tomography (DECT). Eur Radiol 2017;27(4):1622–30.

56. Barrett T, Bowden DJ, Shaida N, et al. Virtual unenhanced second generation dual-source CT of the liver: is it time to discard the conventional unenhanced phase? Eur J Radiol 2012;81(7): 1438–45.

57. Kim YK, Park BK, Kim CK, et al. Adenoma characterization: adrenal protocol with dual-energy CT. Radiology 2013;267(1):155–63.

58. Borhani AA, Kulzer M, Iranpour N, et al. Comparison of true unenhanced and virtual unenhanced (VUE) attenuation values in abdominopelvic single-source rapid kilovoltage-switching spectral CT. Abdom Radiol (NY) 2017;42(3):710–7.

59. Sahni VA, Shinagare AB, Silverman SG. Virtual unenhanced CT images acquired from dual-energy CT urography: accuracy of attenuation values and variation with contrast material phase. Clin Radiol 2013;68(3):264–71.

60. Birnbaum BA, Hindman N, Lee J, et al. Multi-detector row CT attenuation measurements: assessment of intra- and interscanner variability with an anthropomorphic body CT phantom. Radiology 2007; 242(1):109–19.

61. Toepker M, Moritz T, Krauss B, et al. Virtual non-contrast in second-generation, dual-energy computed tomography: reliability of attenuation values. Eur J Radiol 2012;81(3):e398–405.

62. Miller CM, Gupta RT, Paulson EK, et al. Effect of organ enhancement and habitus on estimation of unenhanced attenuation at contrast-enhanced dual-energy MDCT: concepts for individualized and

organ-specific spectral iodine subtraction strategies. AJR Am J Roentgenol 2011;196(5):W558–64.

63. Takahashi N, Hartman RP, Vrtiska TJ, et al. Dual-energy CT iodine-subtraction virtual unenhanced technique to detect urinary stones in an iodine-filled collecting system: a phantom study. AJR Am J Roentgenol 2008;190(5):1169–73.

64. Patel BN, Alexander L, Allen B, et al. Dual-energy CT workflow: multi-institutional consensus on standardization of abdominopelvic MDCT protocols. Abdom Radiol (NY) 2017;42(3):676–87.

65. Botsikas D, Triponez F, Boudabbous S, et al. Incidental adrenal lesions detected on enhanced abdominal dual-energy CT: can the diagnostic workup be shortened by the implementation of virtual unenhanced images? Eur J Radiol 2014; 83(10):1746–51.

66. Kaufmann S, Sauter A, Spira D, et al. Tin-filter enhanced dual-energy-CT: image quality and accuracy of CT numbers in virtual noncontrast imaging. Acad Radiol 2013;20(5):596–603.

67. Krauss B, Grant KL, Schmidt BT, et al. The importance of spectral separation: an assessment of dual-energy spectral separation for quantitative ability and dose efficiency. Invest Radiol 2015; 50(2):114–8.

68. Faby S, Kuchenbecker S, Sawall S, et al. Performance of today's dual energy CT and future multi energy CT in virtual non-contrast imaging and in iodine quantification: a simulation study. Med Phys 2015;42(7):4349–66.

69. Marin D, Mileto A, Gupta RT, et al. Effect of radiologists' experience with an adaptive statistical iterative reconstruction algorithm on detection of hypervascular liver lesions and perception of image quality. Abdom Imaging 2015;40(7):2850–60.

70. Mayo-Smith WW, Song JH, Boland GL, et al. Management of incidental adrenal masses: a white paper of the ACR incidental findings committee. J Am Coll Radiol 2017;14(8):1038–44.

71. Gore RM, Pickhardt PJ, Mortele KJ, et al. Management of incidental liver lesions on CT: a white paper of the ACR incidental findings committee. J Am Coll Radiol 2017;14(11):1429–37.

72. Ho LM, Marin D, Neville AM, et al. Characterization of adrenal nodules with dual-energy CT: can virtual unenhanced attenuation values replace true unenhanced attenuation values? AJR Am J Roentgenol 2012;198(4):840–5.

73. Neville AM, Gupta RT, Miller CM, et al. Detection of renal lesion enhancement with dual-energy multidetector CT. Radiology 2011;259(1):173–83.

74. Song KD, Kim CK, Park BK, et al. Utility of iodine overlay technique and virtual unenhanced images for the characterization of renal masses by dual-energy CT. AJR Am J Roentgenol 2011;197(6): W1076–82.

75. Tian SF, Liu AL, Liu JH, et al. Application of computed tomography virtual noncontrast spectral imaging in evaluation of hepatic metastases: a preliminary study. Chin Med J (Engl) 2015;128(5):610–4.

76. Kim JE, Lee JM, Baek JH, et al. Initial assessment of dual-energy CT in patients with gallstones or bile duct stones: can virtual nonenhanced images replace true nonenhanced images? AJR Am J Roentgenol 2012;198(4):817–24.

77. Lee HA, Lee YH, Yoon KH, et al. Comparison of virtual unenhanced images derived from dual-energy CT with true unenhanced images in evaluation of gallstone disease. AJR Am J Roentgenol 2016; 206(1):74–80.

78. Chen CY, Hsu JS, Jaw TS, et al. Utility of the iodine overlay technique and virtual nonenhanced images for the preoperative T staging of colorectal cancer by dual-energy CT with tin filter technology. PLoS One 2014;9(12):e113589.

79. Sun H, Hou XY, Xue HD, et al. Dual-source dual-energy CT angiography with virtual non-enhanced images and iodine map for active gastrointestinal bleeding: image quality, radiation dose and diagnostic performance. Eur J Radiol 2015;84(5):884–91.

80. Flors L, Leiva-Salinas C, Norton PT, et al. Endoleak detection after endovascular repair of thoracic aortic aneurysm using dual-source dual-energy CT: suitable scanning protocols and potential radiation dose reduction. AJR Am J Roentgenol 2013; 200(2):451–60.

81. Chen CY, Tsai TH, Jaw TS, et al. Diagnostic performance of split-bolus portal venous phase dual-energy CT urography in patients with hematuria. AJR Am J Roentgenol 2016;206(5):1013–22.

82. Wang W, Liu L, Zeng H, et al. Utility of virtual unenhanced images and split-bolus injection using spectral multidetector CT for the assessment of renal cell carcinoma conspicuity and radiation dose. Int J Clin Pract 2016;70(Suppl 9B):B56–63.

83. Brook OR, Gourtsoyianni S, Brook A, et al. Split-bolus spectral multidetector CT of the pancreas: assessment of radiation dose and tumor conspicuity. Radiology 2013;269(1):139–48.

84. Mohammed NM, Mahfouz A, Achkar K, et al. Contrast-induced nephropathy. Heart Views 2013; 14(3):106–16.

85. McDonald RJ, McDonald JS, Newhouse JH, et al. Controversies in contrast material-induced acute kidney injury: closing in on the truth? Radiology 2015;277(3):627–32.

86. Deinzer CK, Danova D, Kleb B, et al. Influence of different iodinated contrast media on the induction of DNA double-strand breaks after in vitro X-ray irradiation. Contrast Media Mol Imaging 2014; 9(4):259–67.

87. Carrascosa P, Capunay C, Rodriguez-Granillo GA, et al. Substantial iodine volume load reduction in CT angiography with dual-energy imaging: insights from a pilot randomized study. Int J Cardiovasc Imaging 2014;30(8):1613–20.

88. Shuman WP, O'Malley RB, Busey JM, et al. Prospective comparison of dual-energy CT aortography using 70% reduced iodine dose versus single-energy CT aortography using standard iodine dose in the same patient. Abdom Radiol (NY) 2017;42(3):759–65.

89. Yu L, Bruesewitz MR, Thomas KB, et al. Optimal tube potential for radiation dose reduction in pediatric CT: principles, clinical implementations, and pitfalls. Radiographics 2011;31(3):835–48.

90. Shen Y, Hu X, Zou X, et al. Did low tube voltage CT combined with low contrast media burden protocols accomplish the goal of "double low" for patients? An overview of applications in vessels and abdominal parenchymal organs over the past 5 years. Int J Clin Pract 2016;70(Suppl 9B):B5–15.

91. Meier A, Wurnig M, Desbiolles L, et al. Advanced virtual monoenergetic images: improving the contrast of dual-energy CT pulmonary angiography. Clin Radiol 2015;70(11):1244–51.

92. Lee JW, Lee G, Lee NK, et al. Effectiveness of adaptive statistical iterative reconstruction for 64-slice dual-energy computed tomography pulmonary angiography in patients with a reduced iodine load: comparison with standard computed tomography pulmonary angiography. J Comput Assist Tomogr 2016;40(5):777–83.

93. Hou P, Feng X, Liu J, et al. Iterative reconstruction in single-source dual-energy CT angiography: feasibility of low and ultra-low volume contrast medium protocols. Br J Radiol 2017;90(1075):20160506.

94. Agrawal MD, Oliveira GR, Kalva SP, et al. Prospective comparison of reduced-iodine-dose virtual monochromatic imaging dataset from dual-energy CT angiography with standard-iodine-dose single-energy CT angiography for abdominal aortic aneurysm. AJR Am J Roentgenol 2016;207(6):W125–32.

95. Shuman WP, Chan KT, Busey JM, et al. Dual-energy CT aortography with 50% reduced iodine dose versus single-energy CT aortography with standard iodine dose. Acad Radiol 2016;23(5):611–8.

96. Iezzi R, Cotroneo AR, Giammarino A, et al. Low-dose multidetector-row CT-angiography of abdominal aortic aneurysm after endovascular repair. Eur J Radiol 2011;79(1):21–8.

97. Goetti R, Winklehner A, Gordic S, et al. Automated attenuation-based kilovoltage selection: preliminary observations in patients after endovascular aneurysm repair of the abdominal aorta. AJR Am J Roentgenol 2012;199(3):W380–5.

98. Ippolito D, Talei Franzesi C, Fior D, et al. Low kV settings CT angiography (CTA) with low dose contrast medium volume protocol in the assessment of thoracic and abdominal aorta disease: a feasibility study. Br J Radiol 2015;88(1049):20140140.

99. Higashigaito K, Schmid T, Puippe G, et al. CT Angiography of the aorta: prospective evaluation of individualized low-volume contrast media protocols. Radiology 2016;280(3):960–8.

100. Nijhof WH, Baltussen EJ, Kant IM, et al. Low-dose CT angiography of the abdominal aorta and reduced contrast medium volume: assessment of image quality and radiation dose. Clin Radiol 2016;71(1):64–73.

101. Xin L, Yang X, Huang N, et al. The initial experience of the upper abdominal CT angiography using low-concentration contrast medium on dual energy spectral CT. Abdom Imaging 2015;40(7):2894–9.

102. He J, Wang Q, Ma X, et al. Dual-energy CT angiography of abdomen with routine concentration contrast agent in comparison with conventional single-energy CT with high concentration contrast agent. Eur J Radiol 2015;84(2):221–7.

103. Meier A, Higashigaito K, Martini K, et al. Dual energy CT pulmonary angiography with 6g iodine-A propensity score-matched study. PLoS One 2016;11(12):e0167214.

104. Almutairi A, Sun Z, Poovathumkadavi A, et al. Dual energy CT angiography of peripheral arterial disease: feasibility of using lower contrast medium volume. PLoS One 2015;10(9):e0139275.

105. Zheng M, Liu Y, Wei M, et al. Low concentration contrast medium for dual-source computed tomography coronary angiography by a combination of iterative reconstruction and low-tube-voltage technique: feasibility study. Eur J Radiol 2014;83(2):e92–9.

106. Mihl C, Wildberger JE, Jurencak T, et al. Intravascular enhancement with identical iodine delivery rate using different iodine contrast media in a circulation phantom. Invest Radiol 2013;48(11):813–8.

107. Liu J, Lv PJ, Wu R, et al. Aortic dual-energy CT angiography with low contrast medium injection rate. J Xray Sci Technol 2014;22(5):689–96.

108. Bae KT. Intravenous contrast medium administration and scan timing at CT: considerations and approaches. Radiology 2010;256(1):32–61.

109. Chung YE, You JS, Lee HJ, et al. Possible contrast media reduction with low keV monoenergetic images in the detection of focal liver lesions: a dual-energy CT animal study. PLoS One 2015;10(7):e0133170.

110. Clark ZE, Bolus DN, Little MD, et al. Abdominal rapid-kVp-switching dual-energy MDCT with reduced IV contrast compared to conventional MDCT with standard weight-based IV contrast: an

intra-patient comparison. Abdom Imaging 2015; 40(4):852–8.

111. Tsang DS, Merchant TE, Merchant SE, et al. Quantifying potential reduction in contrast dose with monoenergetic images synthesized from dual-layer detector spectral CT. Br J Radiol 2017; 90(1078):20170290.

112. Patino M, Murcia DJ, Iamurri AP, et al. Impact of low-energy CT imaging on selection of positive oral contrast media concentration. Abdom Radiol (NY) 2017;42(5):1298–309.

113. Robinson JD, Mitsumori LM, Linnau KF. Evaluating contrast agent waste and costs of weight-based CT contrast bolus protocols using single- or multiple-dose packaging. AJR Am J Roentgenol 2013;200(6):W617–20.

114. Setty BN, Sahani DV, Ouellette-Piazzo K, et al. Comparison of enhancement, image quality, cost, and adverse reactions using 2 different contrast medium concentrations for routine chest CT on 16-slice MDCT. J Comput Assist Tomogr 2006; 30(5):818–22.

Pearls, Pitfalls, and Problems in Dual-Energy Computed Tomography Imaging of the Body

Jeremy R. Wortman, MD*, Aaron D. Sodickson, MD, PhD

KEYWORDS

- Dual-energy CT • Computed tomography • Abdominal imaging • Iodine-selective imaging

KEY POINTS

- Dual-energy computed tomography (DECT) is a disruptive technology that has the potential to change the way that CT is performed and interpreted.
- As the use of DECT grows, it is essential for radiologists to be aware of the fundamental principles of DECT acquisition, postprocessing, and clinical use.
- DECT introduces several unique challenges, imaging artifacts, and potential diagnostic pitfalls that the interpreting radiologist should understand.

INTRODUCTION

Dual-energy computed tomography (DECT) refers to CT acquisition using 2 different x-ray energy spectra, which has the potential to characterize tissues based on their material composition. Although the theoretic possibility of material characterization with DECT has been known since 1976, DECT was not technically feasible with early-generation CT scanners; it was not until the introduction of the first dual-source scanner in 2006 that vendors began to develop DECT technology in earnest. The introduction of DECT has been accompanied by research on a variety of clinical applications in body imaging,[1–8] as well as many technological advancements aimed to increase the use of DECT in routine clinical practice.

As the clinical use of DECT continues to grow, it is important for radiologists to be aware of potential challenges and problems related to performing DECT scans, postprocessing, and displaying images, and incorporating DECT into routine clinical practice. In addition, DECT introduces several unique artifacts and interpretive pitfalls, which may be unfamiliar to radiologists who are new to using this technology.

In this article, we provide a practical overview of DECT in body imaging, focused on problems and diagnostic pitfalls associated with DECT and steps that can be taken to avoid them. Following a review of technical principles and postprocessing techniques available with DECT, we describe several challenges and pitfalls of DECT related to image acquisition, postprocessing and display, and interpretation.

BASIC PRINCIPLES OF DUAL-ENERGY COMPUTED TOMOGRAPHY

With conventional single-energy CT (SECT), imaging is obtained with a single polychromatic energy spectrum, ranging from 80 kVp to

Disclosure Statement: A.D. Sodickson is the principal investigator and J.R. Wortman is a co-investigator on an institutional research grant from Siemens, AG.
Division of Emergency Radiology, Department of Radiology, Brigham and Women's Hospital, Harvard Medical School, 75 Francis Street, Boston, MA 02115, USA
* Corresponding author.
E-mail address: jwortman@bwh.harvard.edu

Radiol Clin N Am 56 (2018) 625–640
https://doi.org/10.1016/j.rcl.2018.03.007
0033-8389/18/© 2018 Elsevier Inc. All rights reserved.

140 kVp depending on the anatomic region and scan indication. DECT instead acquires data with 2 different energy spectra, typically low energy at 80 or 100 kVp and high energy at 140 or 150 kVp. Different vendors have different approaches to DECT data acquisition, including dual-source DECT, which uses 2 different x-ray tubes operating at different kVp, each with a matching detector array; single-source DECT, which rapidly switches between low energy (80 kVp) and high energy (140 kVp) using a single x-ray tube and detector; and dual-layer detector-based DECT, which uses a single 120-kVp x-ray tube, with a layered detector that preferentially absorbs the low-energy or high-energy photons in the superficial and deep detector layers, respectively.

Tissue Differentiation with Dual-Energy Computed Tomography

For materials to be differentiated with DECT, they must have sufficiently different x-ray absorption behaviors as a function of kVp. This is often characterized by the *CT number ratio* of materials, which is defined as the ratio of the CT number (in Hounsfield units [HU]) of the material at low energy to the CT number of the same material at high energy.[9] For example, iodine and calcium both exhibit higher HU values at low kVp compared with high kVp, with iodine having a higher CT number ratio than calcium (**Fig. 1**) due to its greater atomic number and its k-edge near the mean of the low-kVp energy

spectrum. Conversely, fat and uric acid demonstrate lower HU values as kVp increases. Most other soft tissues behave similarly at high and low kVp, and thus have CT number ratios close to 1.

The difference between CT number ratios of materials is determined not only by the atomic number of the materials, but also by the *spectral separation* between the low-energy and high-energy spectra. The greater the separation between the 2 energy spectra, the easier it is to distinguish between materials with DECT. Unfortunately, there is a large degree of spectral overlap between the typical high-energy and low-energy spectra, and methods to increase spectral separation are thus crucial to tissue differentiation with DECT. A variety of techniques have been used to increase spectral separation: adding a tin (Sn) filter in front of the high-energy x-ray tube on dual-source systems to preferentially attenuate the low-energy photons in the spectrum, or using the highest possible difference between kVp values, including use of 80 kVp for the low-energy spectrum, or still lower kVp values when available on the scanner.[9,10]

Dual-Energy Computed Tomography Postprocessing

For each dual-energy acquisition, an image series is typically sent to the Picture Archive and Communication System (PACS) for routine interpretation that is a weighted average of the high and low-energy data. This is commonly referred

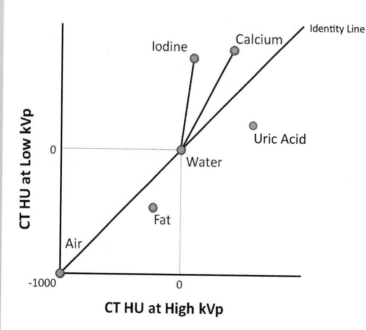

Fig. 1. Material-dependent x-ray absorption with DECT. HU values of different materials exposed to low kVp (y axis) and high kVp (x axis) x-ray spectra. Water and air are calibrated to 0 and −1000 HU, respectively. Iodine and calcium show progressively higher x-ray absorption at low energy, with characteristic slopes as concentration increases. Fat and uric acid demonstrate lower x-ray absorption as x-ray energy is decreased. Most other soft tissues lie very close to the identity line.

to as a *mixed* or *blended* dataset, and is intended to have an image appearance similar to a conventional 120-kVp single-energy scan. Blending the 2 datasets combines the benefits of the increased contrast of the low-energy data with the decreased noise of the high-energy data.

There are many imaging display types available with DECT postprocessing. Materials that are differentiated or quantified using DECT can be displayed with the use of *material-specific images*. Single-source systems create these images using a 2-material decomposition algorithm, whereby each voxel is decomposed into the expected behavior of 2 basis set materials (typically iodine and water or the photoelectric and Compton scatter effects), which may then be blended in different combinations to create the material map of interest. Dual-source systems typically create these images using a 3-material decomposition algorithm, whereby each voxel is assumed to be composed of a mixture of 3 materials (often iodine, fat, and soft tissue for most abdominal applications), and the contribution of each material is calculated based on the known x-ray absorption behavior of each material.

Several different variations of material-specific imaging can be performed and displayed. With *iodine-selective imaging*, the principle of material decomposition is used to selectively image iodine. Iodine can be subtracted from an image, creating a virtual noncontrast (VNC) image (**Fig. 2**). Alternatively, iodine content can be visualized directly

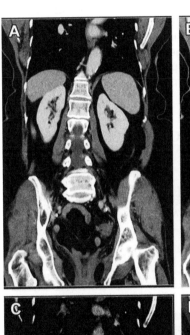
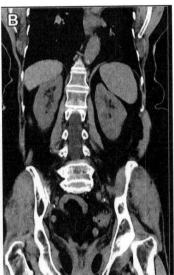
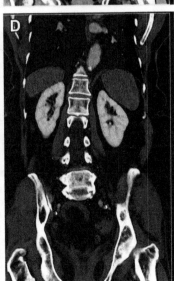

Fig. 2. Iodine-selective imaging with DECT. Iodine can be subtracted from the initial mixed image (*A*), which creates a VNC image (*B*). Conversely, iodine can be selectively displayed in a color-coded iodine map (*C*). Superimposing the iodine map on top of the grayscale VNC image yields an iodine overlay image (*D*), which provides increased anatomic detail.

with color-coded iodine images, either in the form of iodine maps or iodine overlay images that display the iodine content superimposed on a grayscale VNC image. In our experience, readers prefer the iodine overlay image to the iodine map, as it provides information regarding iodine content in color with greater underlying grayscale anatomic detail for localization. Color-coded iodine images can be used both for qualitative and quantitative assessments of iodine enhancement.

Several other material-specific imaging displays are available with DECT. If calcium is subtracted from images rather than iodine, *virtual noncalcium* images can be created in which the trabecular bone is removed from images, which allows bone marrow edema to be visualized. Similarly, for vascular imaging, bones can be removed to improve maximum intensity projection images and better visualize vessels traversing osseous foramina, and calcified plaque can be subtracted from images, potentially improving assessment of vasculature with heavily calcified plaques.

Another postprocessing display available with DECT is *virtual monoenergetic imaging* (VMI). With all CT imaging, data are acquired using a polychromatic energy spectrum. VMI can be derived from dual-energy acquisitions, and create simulated images as if the scan had been obtained at a single energy level (keV), allowing the user to manipulate the keV (**Fig. 3**). This has a variety of potential applications, including increasing iodine contrast with low-keV images, reducing beam hardening artifact with high-keV images, and many others.[11]

CHALLENGES, PROBLEMS, AND DIAGNOSTIC PITFALLS WITH DUAL-ENERGY COMPUTED TOMOGRAPHY

In the following sections, we review potential challenges, artifacts, and diagnostic pitfalls associated with DECT, and how they can be overcome. We separate these into 3 broad categories: image acquisition, image artifacts and limitations associated with DECT postprocessed images, and specific interpretive pitfalls.

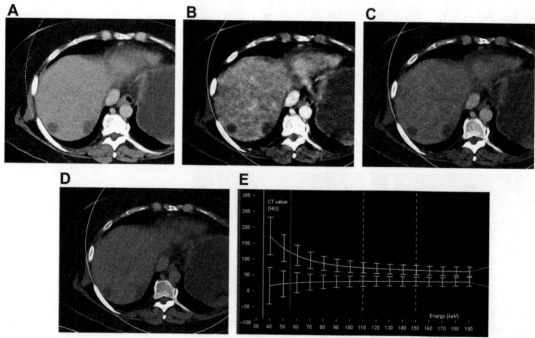

Fig. 3. A 68-year-old woman with metastatic colorectal cancer. The patient's liver metastases are visible on the mixed image (*A*). Virtual monoenergetic images were reconstructed at 40 keV (*B*), 60 keV (*C*), and 130 keV (*D*). The contrast between the metastases and the liver parenchyma is greatest at 40 keV; however, noise is also greatest on this image. At 60 keV, the lesions are more conspicuous than on the mixed image, with decreased noise compared with 40 keV. At high (130) keV, the contrast of the lesions is decreased. Virtual monoenergetic curves (*E*) of a lesion (*white curve*) and liver parenchyma (*yellow curve*) provide a graphical representation of the difference in HU between the liver and the metastases at different keV values, with the error bars representing image noise.

IMAGE ACQUISITION
Radiation Dose Concerns

Concerns regarding radiation dose of DECT are common, but are largely based on a misconception that because DECT acquires data at 2 different energy levels, it will have a higher radiation dose than SECT. However, in clinical practice, DECT is performed by dividing the radiation dose of the scan between the high-energy and low-energy acquisitions. DECT protocols can therefore be designed to be of equivalent or lower dose when compared with SECT protocols, with preserved image quality. This has been demonstrated with abdominal CT,[12] pediatric thoracic and abdominal CT,[13] CT pulmonary angiography,[14] abdominal CT angiography,[15] and a variety of other practice settings.

In addition, there are many opportunities for radiation dose reduction with DECT. Perhaps the greatest potential to reduce dose with DECT is by using VNC images to replace a separate noncontrast acquisition in multiphase protocols, thus eliminating an entire scan phase and substantially decreasing the overall dose of the scan. The ability to reduce dose by replacing an unenhanced acquisition with a VNC acquisition has been used in many clinical settings, including renal mass protocol CT,[1] CT urography,[16] adrenal washout CT,[17] CT angiography for gastrointestinal (GI) bleeding,[18,19] and multiphase liver CT.[20]

Another method by which DECT can reduce radiation dose is in the characterization of incidental lesions; DECT has been validated in assessing these lesions, most notably within the kidneys and adrenal glands.[21] By definitively characterizing such lesions at the time of their initial detection, unnecessary follow-up imaging can be avoided, further decreasing overall radiation dose to the patient.

Field of View

On dual-source systems, the high-energy detector has a smaller field of view than the low-energy detector (either 26 cm, 33 cm, or 35 cm depending on the generation of scanner). Particularly for a patient who is poorly centered in the scanner gantry, this can result in peripheral patient anatomy being excluded from dual-energy acquisition. Anatomy outside of the dual-energy field of view will also have degraded image quality on mixed images, as it will appear as if it is imaged only by the low-energy spectrum. This is most commonly an issue in large patients in whom significant portions of anatomy may be excluded from the dual-energy acquisition, and trauma patients who are difficult to position centrally within the gantry (**Fig. 4**). Although this limitation cannot be completely overcome, it can be mitigated by educating CT technologists as to the importance of carefully centering patients, and taking care to include any anatomy that is known (before the scan) to need dual-energy characterization within the dual-energy field of view.

ARTIFACTS AND LIMITATIONS ASSOCIATED WITH DUAL-ENERGY COMPUTED TOMOGRAPHY POSTPROCESSED IMAGES
Photon Starvation, Beam Hardening, and Metal Artifact

Photon starvation, beam hardening, and metal artifact present unique challenges with DECT imaging, due to the limited beam penetration of low-energy photons. This can cause problems in imaging large patients (particularly in abdomen/pelvis CT), trauma patients (who may require their arms to be positioned down during the scan), and all patients with metallic hardware. In addition, this poses challenges in imaging the neck and cervical

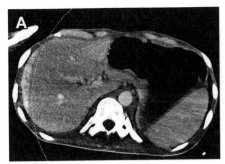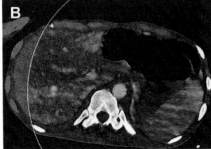

Fig. 4. A 32-year-old male patient with contrast-enhanced DECT poorly centered within the gantry. On the axial mixed images (*A*), the periphery of the liver is outside of the smaller field of view, and thus appears hyperattenuating as it is only imaged by the 80 kVp spectrum. On the axial iodine overlay images (*B*), iodine content cannot be assessed from the anatomy outside of the dual energy field of view.

spine, due to photon starvation from the shoulders.

Beam hardening and photon starvation are more likely at low kVp, and thus these artifacts are more likely to occur if 80 kVp is used for the low-energy acquisition.[22] On fast kV switching single-source systems, 80 kVp and 140 kVp pairs are the only option, leading many radiologists to limit DECT acquisition only to smaller patients (often <260–280 pounds) because 80 kVp photon starvation markedly impairs DECT image quality for larger patients.[23] As an alternative, dual-source systems use a tin filter in front of the high-energy (140 or 150 kVp) source to improve spectral separation, which enables acquisition using a 100-kVp low-energy source in larger patients to overcome photon starvation effects.[10]

In addition to significantly degrading image quality on mixed images, these artifacts can cause errors on DECT postprocessed images. On color-coded iodine images, streak artifact can create the false appearance of either an excessive amount or a lack of iodine content (Fig. 5), rendering these images nondiagnostic. This is a particular challenge with perfused blood volume maps on CT pulmonary angiograms, as artifact from dense contrast in the superior vena cava is common. Similarly, photon starvation and beam hardening can lead to inaccuracies on color-coded iodine images in large patients, particularly within centrally located anatomy (Fig. 6). These artifacts also can lead to inaccurate assessment of renal stones; because renal stone characterization depends on the CT number ratio of the stone (to distinguish calcium-based from uric acid stones), errors in the HU measurements caused by these artifacts can cause stones to be misclassified (Fig. 7).

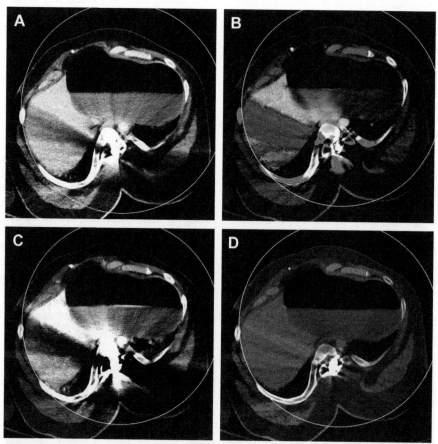

Fig. 5. Example of the impact of metal artifact on DECT postprocessed images. On the axial mixed image (*A*), streak artifact from the patient's spinal hardware degrades image quality in the liver. On the corresponding iodine overlay image (*B*), there is the false appearance of complete lack of iodine content within this region of the liver, and erroneously increased iodine content close to the metal. This artifact is accentuated on a low (40) keV virtual monoenergetic image (*C*), and decreases at high (190) keV (*D*), although iodine content is also suppressed due to the high keV.

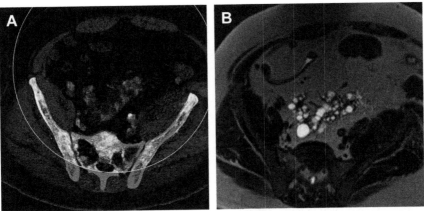

Fig. 6. Axial iodine overlay image (A) in a patient with a horseshoe kidney with multiple renal cysts. Many of these cysts appear to have color-coded iodine content within them. On the subsequently obtained MR image, the T2-weighted image (B) demonstrates that these predominantly represent simple cysts. The appearance of iodine content is artifactual due to noise and central location of the horseshoe kidney.

There are many tools that can be used to help resolve these artifacts. Virtual monoenergetic images can be used to mitigate against beam hardening artifact (and the contribution of beam hardening to metal artifact), particularly at high keV.[24] However, at high keV, iodine contrast is also suppressed (see Fig. 5), limiting the clinical utility of these images for contrast-enhanced or CT angiogram applications. In addition, virtual monoenergetic images have several other limitations in metal artifact reduction. Reduction of metal artifact at high keV is highly dependent on the quantity, configuration, and type of metal. In addition, high-keV images provide no benefit in regions suffering from photon starvation. Instead, better image quality improvements are typically found in such areas using available metal artifact reduction algorithms that can be applied either to SECT or DECT (see Fig. 7).

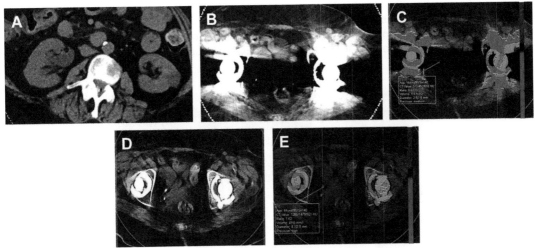

Fig. 7. Inaccurate stone characterization due to artifact. This 68-year-old woman with a history of nephrolithiasis and prior bilateral hip replacements presented with right flank pain. Axial image at the level of the kidneys (A) demonstrates mild right hydronephrosis, due to an obstructing right distal ureteral stone (B), difficult to visualize due to streak artifact from the patient's hip prostheses. This artifact, which is greater at low kVp, results in incorrect characterization of the stone as uric acid, color-coded red on the stone overlay image (C). When projection-based iterative metal artifact reduction is applied to the low and high kVp source images, not only do the stones become more apparent on the mixed image (D), but the stone is then correctly characterized as calcium and is color-coded in blue on the subsequently reconstructed stone overlay image (E), in keeping with the patient's other nonobstructing renal stones (not shown).

On dual-source systems, photon starvation and beam hardening can be reduced by using 100 kVp for the low-energy acquisition to improve beam penetration. At our institution, for abdominal DECT, all trauma patients are imaged at 100/Sn140kVp to improve image quality for spine reconstructions (**Fig. 8**).[25] For nontrauma patients, most patients are imaged at 80/Sn140kVp, with the exception of patients with an anteroposterior diameter greater than 33 cm on the lateral planning radiograph (the size of the smaller field of view on second-generation dual-source DECT scanners), in whom our technologists switch to 100/Sn140kVp. We have found that this approach is able to maintain image quality in large patients, and allows for diagnostic-quality spine reformats in the trauma setting.

Image Noise on Virtual Monoenergetic Images

Although there are a myriad of clinical uses for virtual monoenergetic images, one of the inherent problems with these images is the increased noise associated with the extremes of low and high keV. Because of this, some of the studies demonstrating clinical benefit of these images have also documented decreases in subjective image quality and increases in image noise.[26] Vendors have worked to solve this problem, primarily by developing a second-generation monoenergetic algorithm that significantly reduces image noise[27] (Monoenergetic Plus; Siemens Healthcare, Forchheim, Germany). This was developed using a frequency split technique that uses the high-contrast data from low-keV images for low spatial frequencies (object information),

and combines this with the lower noise data at higher keV (near 70 keV) for higher spatial frequencies to reduce noise and improve image quality.

Display Settings and Noise of Color-Coded Iodine Images

To accurately evaluate for iodine content, color-coded iodine images must have appropriate window and level settings. If the window/level settings are incorrect, it will create the appearance of iodine content within structures that should not contain iodine, such as air or subcutaneous fat. This can create the false impression that iodine is present within lesions that do not contain iodine, such as simple renal cysts (**Fig. 9**). When interpreting these images, it is important to adjust these settings so that there is no color-coded iodine within structures that would not be expected to contain iodine, and the iodine content of the organs and vasculature is easily visualized.

Even with appropriate window and level settings, there is some inherent noise present on color-coded iodine images that can confound interpretation. Noise on iodine overlay images can create the appearance of faint iodine content within lesions that do not contain iodine (**Fig. 10**). This may be caused by a variety of factors, including inherent noise within the algorithms used to calculate iodine concentration, as well as the scan technique and radiation dose.

Limitations of Iodine Quantification

There are many inherent limitations in using DECT to quantify the iodine content. Although

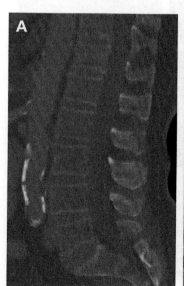 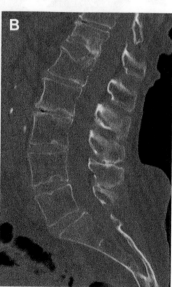

Fig. 8. Example of spine reformats in 2 different large patients. Image (*A*) was acquired at 80/Sn140 kVp, whereas image (*B*) was acquired at 100/Sn140 kVp. Image quality is significantly improved using 100/Sn140 kVp as a result of the improved penetration of the low-energy beam at 100 kVp.

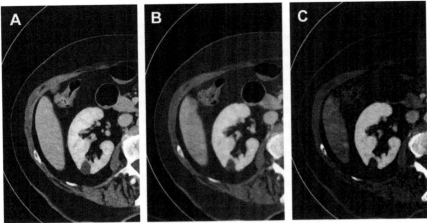

Fig. 9. Appropriate and inappropriate window and level settings on color-coded iodine images. On the axial mixed image (*A*), there is a small simple renal cyst in the interpolar right kidney, which measures fluid attenuation. An iodine overlay image with incorrect window and level settings (*B*) demonstrates the false impression that there is color-coded iodine content within this simple cyst. There is also color-coded iodine content within the air and subcutaneous fat, an indication that windowing is incorrect. Once the iodine overlay image is windowed correctly (*C*), it becomes clear that there is no iodine content within this simple cyst. At our institution, we use a width of 150 and center of 80 for the iodine color overlay display.

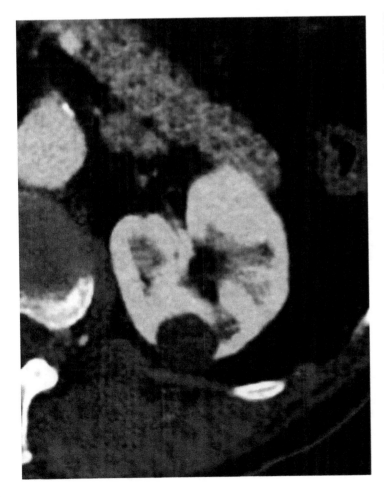

Fig. 10. Axial iodine overlay image in a patient with a known simple renal cyst. Some faint orange can be seen within the cyst, an example of noise causing the false appearance of iodine content.

the iodine concentration can be measured within lesions, there are no well-validated thresholds to truly distinguish between enhancing and nonenhancing lesions. Many individual studies in the literature have reported possible thresholds for renal lesions[28–30]; however, the numbers reported are variable, and there is likely to be significant variation between different vendor platforms. Although there is a similar limitation to using fixed HU enhancement thresholds with SECT (eg, 10–20 HU), the thresholds used with SECT have been better established in the literature. More research is needed to establish well-validated thresholds with DECT to define true enhancement, and to ensure that these thresholds are generalizable between vendors.

Another inherent limitation to iodine quantification with DECT is the ability to measure noise. Although measurements of iodine enhancement can be performed with DECT, the standard deviation measurements of iodine enhancement do not truly reflect image noise in the traditional sense, as they incorporate systematic errors within the algorithm as well. In addition, vendor platforms do not provide standard deviation measurements for iodine concentration measurements, which can make these measurements harder to interpret.

An additional limitation of iodine quantification with DECT is that when color-coded iodine images are sent to PACS, these images cannot be used for quantitative assessment, as Digital Imaging and Communication in Medicine (DICOM) standard cannot yet process HU measurements on color images. Because of this, when these images are sent to PACS, only qualitative assessment can

be made; quantitative analysis requires either sending grayscale iodine images to PACS, or for the radiologist to evaluate images in vendor software.

Incomplete Iodine Subtraction

When extremely high concentrations of iodine are present (eg, bright arterial boluses, dense iodinated enteric contrast within bowel loops, concentrated contrast within the renal collecting systems), subtraction of iodine may be incomplete on VNC images, with residual iodine present (Fig. 11). This can confound assessment of virtual noncontrast images in some patients, and may particularly be an important limitation of iodine-selective imaging in vascular studies, as the presence of residual contrast within the lumen on VNC images could mask or mimic pathology.

SPECIFIC INTERPRETATIVE CHALLENGES AND PITFALLS
Distinguishing Iodine from Other Dense Materials

One benefit of iodine-selective imaging is the ability to distinguish iodine from other dense materials on a single-phase contrast-enhanced DECT scan. This can be helpful in a number of clinical scenarios: distinguishing between ingested material within the bowel lumen (eg, bismuth) and active GI bleeding (Fig. 12); differentiating hematoma from iodine enhancement; and in trauma patients, distinguishing bone fragments from contrast extravasation.

When using iodine-selective images to distinguish iodine from other dense materials, it is crucial to always review both VNC and color-coded iodine

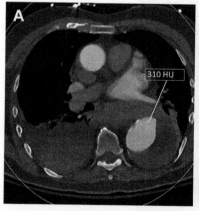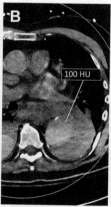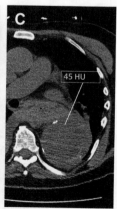

Fig. 11. A 58-year-old man with dissection of the descending thoracic aorta, with rupture into the pleural space. The dense contrast (310 HU) within the true lumen of the descending thoracic aorta (A) is incompletely subtracted on the virtual noncontrast image (B), where it measures 100 HU, and would thus be expected to mask adjacent intramural hematoma if it were present. The same area on a true noncontrast image (C) measures 45 HU.

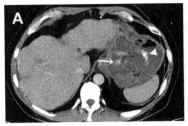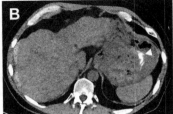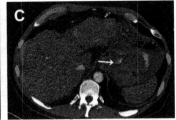

Fig. 12. DECT in a 50-year-old man with hematemesis. On the mixed image (*A*), there are several foci of high-attenuation material within the stomach (*arrow, arrowhead*). On the VNC image (*B*), one of these foci persists (*arrowhead*), indicating that this represents ingested material, likely bismuth. The other focus disappears on the VNC image and contains color-coded iodine content on the iodine overlay image (*C, arrow*), consistent with a site of active bleeding.

images together. Many intrinsically dense materials (eg, bismuth) appear bright on VNC images, without associated color-coded iodine content on iodine maps or overlay images. However, calcium has a unique appearance on these images; using 3-material decomposition algorithms, calcium is decomposed into both VNC and iodine components, and thus will remain bright on both VNC and color-coded iodine images (**Fig. 13**). If color-coded iodine images are interpreted in isolation without viewing the corresponding VNC image, calcium can be confused for iodine content, causing errors in interpretation.

Conversely, another potential pitfall is that both iodinated and barium-containing enteric contrast materials are similarly subtracted out from VNC images due to their nearly identical energy-dependent x-ray absorption behaviors. Thus, if a small volume of iodine-containing material is detected incidentally within a bowel loop, it may be difficult or impossible to tell if this represents previously ingested enteric contrast or GI bleeding. However, in most cases the clinical presentation and patient history will be able to differentiate between these 2 entities.

Renal Mass Characterization

One of the most robustly validated applications of DECT is the assessment of renal masses, primarily with iodine-selective imaging. DECT has demonstrated accuracy in distinguishing enhancing from nonenhancing masses, evaluating complex cystic renal masses, and distinguishing between subtypes of renal cell carcinoma.[29–33] For dedicated renal mass evaluation, VNC images are

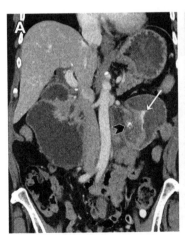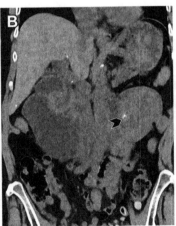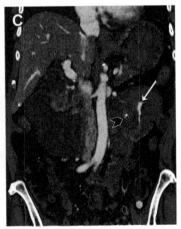

Fig. 13. An 80-year-old woman with jejunal carcinoma. On the coronal mixed image (*A*), there is a jejunal mass with internal calcifications (*arrowhead*). In addition, there is hyperdense material within an adjacent jejunal loop (*arrow*). On the corresponding VNC image (*B*), the calcifications within the mass remain bright (*arrowhead*); however, the hyperdense material within the adjacent bowel loop is not seen, indicating that this material contains iodine and represents a site of active GI bleeding. On the iodine overlay image (*C*), the calcifications (*arrowhead*) within the mass and the site of GI bleeding (*arrow*) both appear bright; if these were interpreted in isolation, the calcifications could be falsely interpreted as an additional site of hemorrhage.

reliable in assessment of the unenhanced attenuation of renal lesions, and enhancement values obtained with single-phase DECT are as reliable as those obtained from multiphase examinations.[28,34,35]

There are several pitfalls that an interpreting radiologist must be aware of when using iodine-selective images to evaluate a renal mass. Occasionally, simple renal cysts will exhibit an increase in attenuation on CT, which has been termed "pseudoenhancement." This occurs most commonly with cysts smaller than 2 cm, and is more likely to occur when imaging is performed at the time of peak parenchymal enhancement. The presence of pseudoenhancement can create a challenge when interpreting color-coded iodine images, as a pseudoenhancing simple renal cyst will falsely appear to have iodine content on these images, and the use of these images may make this pseudoenhancement more conspicuous (Fig. 14).

There are potential remedies offered by DECT to the problem of pseudoenhancement. Virtual monoenergetic images have been demonstrated to reduce renal cyst pseudoenhancement, likely due to the decrease in beam hardening artifact (which contributes to pseudoenhancement). This has been best demonstrated at high keV; studies have shown a substantial reduction in pseudoenhancement using VMI at ranges from 70 to 140 keV (see Fig. 14).[36,37]

The presence of calcifications within a renal mass can also cause interpretive errors with DECT. Calcifications within renal lesions are common, and the presence of nodular or thick calcifications within a cystic lesion is an indication to obtain follow-up imaging. As was mentioned in the prior section, calcium appears bright on both virtual noncontrast and color-coded iodine images. If color-coded iodine images are interpreted in isolation, this can lead to mischaracterization of calcium as iodine enhancement (Fig. 15).

Renal Stone Characterization

CT is an excellent test for evaluation of flank pain and obstructive uropathy caused by urolithiasis, and provides valuable information about stone burden, degree of obstruction, and size and

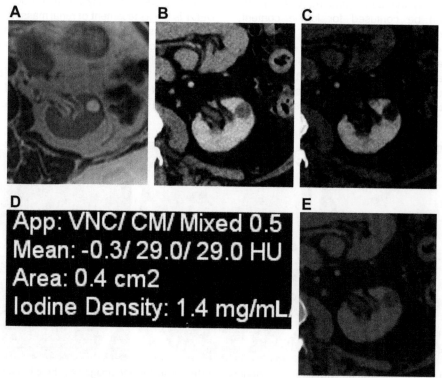

Fig. 14. An 80-year-old woman with pseudoenhancing simple renal cyst. Patient with a simple renal cyst confirmed on MR imaging (representative T2-weighted image shown in [A]). The cyst is hyperattenuating (measuring 29 HU) on mixed images (B), and appears to demonstrate color-coded iodine content (C). Quantitative analysis of the cyst (D) shows 29 HU of enhancement (due to contrast media [CM]), with an iodine concentration of 1.4 mg/mL. On 100 keV virtual monoenergetic images (E), pseudoenhancement decreases, with the cyst measuring 12 HU.

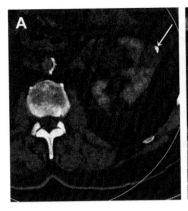 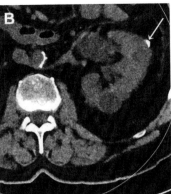

Fig. 15. Calcifications within a renal cyst with DECT. On the axial iodine overlay image (*A*), there is a left interpolar renal lesion with a peripheral focus that appears bright (*arrow*). The corresponding virtual noncontrast image (*B*) demonstrates that this represents intrinsically hyperdense calcification (*arrow*). Note that the vertebral body and calcifications within the abdominal aorta also appear bright on the iodine overlay image.

location of ureteral stones. SECT cannot, however, accurately determine the chemical composition of a renal stone. Most urinary stones are of calcium-based composition, which can be removed when necessary only by invasive interventional urinary procedures or shock wave lithotripsy. However, 5% to 10% of urinary stones are composed of uric acid, which can be gradually dissolved by alkalinizing the urine. Because uric acid has the unique property of exhibiting lower HU values at lower kVp, unlike calcium, which exhibits a marked increase in HU at lower kVp, DECT can accurately differentiate uric acid from calcium-based stones, with direct implications for subsequent management.[38–40]

There are several potential pitfalls to consider in DECT renal stone assessment. Accurate renal stone assessment depends on evaluation of the CT number ratio of the stone, to determine if it is calcium based or uric acid based. As was discussed previously, if there is extensive beam hardening artifact present, this may impact the HU measurements of the stone, particularly at low energy, and thus cause stones to be misclassified (see **Fig. 7**). Similarly, evaluation of stone composition in large patients can be limited due to noise, particularly in stones smaller than 3 mm, decreasing accuracy in this subset of patients.[41] Another potential pitfall of stone assessment with DECT occurs when analyzing VNC images. Because calcium is decomposed equally into VNC and iodine images, small stones at the limits of detectability can theoretically disappear on VNC images if these are used to optimize stone detection from a postcontrast CT (eg, if the noncontrast acquisition is eliminated from a renal mass protocol CT or a CT urogram).

Adrenal Mass Characterization

Adrenal mass characterization is another established clinical application of DECT. On conventional CT, a homogeneous adrenal lesion can be reliably diagnosed as a lipid-rich adenoma if it has an unenhanced attenuation of less than 10 HU.[42] For masses with attenuation of greater than 10 HU on contrast-enhanced DECT, VNC images can be used to measure unenhanced attenuation, and possibly exonerate some lesions as lipid-rich adenomas.

Most studies have shown that attenuation measurements on VNC images are equivalent to traditional noncontrast images.[17,43,44] However, some studies have found that VNC attenuation measurements slightly overestimate the true unenhanced attenuation of adrenal lesions.[45,46] This could present a problem by decreasing sensitivity of diagnosis in cases with borderline attenuation, whereby lipid-rich adenomas that would measure below 10 HU on true noncontrast images may measure slightly above 10 HU on VNC images. Although this would decrease sensitivity in diagnosis with VNC images, the specificity would not change, and this high specificity is essential to ensure there are no false-negative results.

An additional limitation of adrenal mass characterization with DECT is that direct measurements of attenuation on VNC images are not possible with some vendors. In these cases, as a substitute for VNC images, high-energy (eg, 140 keV) virtual monoenergetic images can be used as an alternative means of suppressing iodine content, and creating HU values close to those of a noncontrast image, which may be able to characterize some lesions as lipid-rich adenomas. However, this limitation is also likely to decrease the sensitivity for diagnosis with these vendor platforms.

Liver and Pancreatic Mass Detection and Characterization

Detection of small liver or pancreatic lesions is often challenging with CT, due to the limited contrast between these lesions and the surrounding liver parenchyma. With DECT, viewing low-keV virtual monoenergetic images or low-kVp source images can increase enhancement differences between hypovascular or hypervascular tumors and the surrounding organ parenchyma, which can be helpful in both the liver and the pancreas. Using low-keV/kVp images has been well-validated in improving contrast-to-noise ratio of liver lesions,[26,47–49] and in evaluation of pancreatic adenocarcinoma.[50,51]

The largest challenge in using low-keV monoenergetic images in assessing small lesions is selecting the optimal keV level, to balance the increased contrast at low keV with the inherently increased noise of these images. The optimal keV level depends on a variety of factors, including the generation of software used to reconstruct monoenergetic images, the noise of the scan, and the vascularity of the tumor. In general, studies using first-generation software to create VMI showed optimal keV levels near 70 keV in evaluation of liver and pancreatic lesions,[52,53] while those using second-generation software showed optimal keV levels closer to 50 keV.[54] To visually evaluate for the optimal keV level to maximize lesion contrast, some software packages allow users to create graphical representations of the HU values (and noise levels) of different structures at different keV levels (see **Fig. 3**). Evaluating these graphs for a liver lesion and the liver parenchyma allows a user to select the keV that maximizes the contrast between these 2 structures while minimizing noise.

SUMMARY

DECT is a technology that has the potential to change how CT is performed and interpreted. As more institutions acquire scanners with dual-energy capability, it is crucial for radiologists to be aware of the basic principles and clinical applications of DECT, possible problems and challenges with DECT acquisition, as well as the pitfalls and artifacts that are unique to DECT. Continued work is needed to mitigate these pitfalls, further define the clinical realms in which DECT can add value, and develop workflow solutions that allow this technology to gain more routine clinical use.

REFERENCES

1. Graser A, Johnson TR, Hecht EM, et al. Dual-energy CT in patients suspected of having renal masses: can virtual nonenhanced images replace true nonenhanced images? Radiology 2009;252(2):433–40.

2. Abbara S, Sahani D. Dual-energy computed tomography: promised land or empty promise? J Cardiovasc Comput Tomogr 2008;2(4):243–4.

3. Fletcher JG, Takahashi N, Hartman R, et al. Dual-energy and dual-source CT: is there a role in the abdomen and pelvis? Radiol Clin North Am 2009; 47(1):41–57.

4. Macari M, Spieler B, Kim D, et al. Dual-source dual-energy MDCT of pancreatic adenocarcinoma: initial observations with data generated at 80 kVp and at simulated weighted-average 120 kVp. Am J Roentgenol 2010;194(1):W27–32.

5. Graser A, Johnson TRC, Chandarana H, et al. Dual energy CT: preliminary observations and potential clinical applications in the abdomen. Eur Radiol 2009;19(1):13–23.

6. Thomas C, Patschan O, Ketelsen D, et al. Dual-energy CT for the characterization of urinary calculi: in vitro and in vivo evaluation of a low-dose scanning protocol. Eur Radiol 2009;19(6):1553.

7. Boll DT, Patil NA, Paulson EK, et al. Renal stone assessment with dual-energy multidetector CT and advanced postprocessing techniques: improved characterization of renal stone composition—pilot study. Radiology 2009;250(3):813–20.

8. Stolzmann P, Frauenfelder T, Pfammatter T, et al. Endoleaks after endovascular abdominal aortic aneurysm repair: detection with dual-energy dual-source CT. Radiology 2008;249(2):682–91.

9. Primak AN, Ramirez Giraldo JC, Liu X, et al. Improved dual-energy material discrimination for dual-source CT by means of additional spectral filtration. Med Phys 2009;36(4):1359–69.

10. Krauss B, Grant KL, Schmidt BT, et al. The importance of spectral separation: an assessment of dual-energy spectral separation for quantitative ability and dose efficiency. Invest Radiol 2015;50(2): 114–8.

11. Marin D, Boll DT, Mileto A, et al. State of the art: dual-energy CT of the abdomen. Radiology 2014;271(2): 327–42.

12. Purysko AS, Primak AN, Baker ME, et al. Comparison of radiation dose and image quality from single-energy and dual-energy CT examinations in the same patients screened for hepatocellular carcinoma. Clin Radiol 2014;69(12):e538–44.

13. Siegel MJ, Curtis WA, Ramirez-Giraldo JC. Effects of dual-energy technique on radiation exposure and image quality in pediatric body CT. Am J Roentgenol 2016;207(4):826–35.

14. Zordo TD, von Lutterotti K, Dejaco C, et al. Comparison of image quality and radiation dose of different pulmonary CTA protocols on a 128-slice CT: high-pitch dual source CT, dual energy CT and conventional spiral CT. Eur Radiol 2012;22(2):279–86.

15. Pinho DF, Kulkarni NM, Krishnaraj A, et al. Initial experience with single-source dual-energy CT

abdominal angiography and comparison with single-energy CT angiography: image quality, enhancement, diagnosis and radiation dose. Eur Radiol 2013;23(2):351–9.

16. Ascenti G, Mileto A, Gaeta M, et al. Single-phase dual-energy CT urography in the evaluation of haematuria. Clin Radiol 2013;68(2):e87–94.

17. Ho LM, Marin D, Neville AM, et al. Characterization of adrenal nodules with dual-energy CT: can virtual unenhanced attenuation values replace true unenhanced attenuation values? Am J Roentgenol 2012;198(4):840–5.

18. Sun H, Hou X-Y, Xue H-D, et al. Dual-source dual-energy CT angiography with virtual non-enhanced images and iodine map for active gastrointestinal bleeding: image quality, radiation dose and diagnostic performance. Eur J Radiol 2015;84(5):884–91.

19. Sun H, Xue H-D, Wang Y-N, et al. Dual-source dual-energy computed tomography angiography for active gastrointestinal bleeding: a preliminary study. Clin Radiol 2013;68(2):139–47.

20. Zhang L-J, Peng J, Wu S-Y, et al. Liver virtual non-enhanced CT with dual-source, dual-energy CT: a preliminary study. Eur Radiol 2010;20(9):2257–64.

21. Wortman JR, Bunch PM, Fulwadhva UP, et al. Dual-energy CT of incidental findings in the abdomen: can we reduce the need for follow-up imaging? AJR Am J Roentgenol 2016;W1–11.

22. Guimarães LS, Fletcher JG, Harmsen WS, et al. Appropriate patient selection at abdominal dual-energy CT using 80 kV: relationship between patient size, image noise, and image quality. Radiology 2010;257(3):732–42.

23. Patel BN, Alexander L, Allen B, et al. Dual-energy CT workflow: multi-institutional consensus on standardization of abdominopelvic MDCT protocols. Abdom Radiol (NY) 2017;42(3):676–87.

24. Bamberg F, Dierks A, Nikolaou K, et al. Metal artifact reduction by dual energy computed tomography using monoenergetic extrapolation. Eur Radiol 2011;21(7):1424–9.

25. Wortman JR, Uyeda JW, Fulwadhva UP, et al. Dual energy CT for abdominal and pelvic trauma. Radiographics 2011;38(2):586–602.

26. Altenbernd J, Heusner TA, Ringelstein A, et al. Dual-energy-CT of hypervascular liver lesions in patients with HCC: investigation of image quality and sensitivity. Eur Radiol 2011;21(4):738–43.

27. Grant KL, Flohr TG, Krauss B, et al. Assessment of an advanced image-based technique to calculate virtual monoenergetic computed tomographic images from a dual-energy examination to improve contrast-to-noise ratio in examinations using iodinated contrast media. Invest Radiol 2014;49(9):586–92.

28. Kaza RK, Caoili EM, Cohan RH, et al. Distinguishing enhancing from nonenhancing renal lesions with fast kilovoltage-switching dual-energy CT. Am J Roentgenol 2011;197(6):1375–81.

29. Mileto A, Marin D, Alfaro-Cordoba M, et al. Iodine quantification to distinguish clear cell from papillary renal cell carcinoma at dual-energy multidetector CT: a multireader diagnostic performance study. Radiology 2014;273(3):813–20.

30. Ascenti G, Mileto A, Krauss B, et al. Distinguishing enhancing from nonenhancing renal masses with dual-source dual-energy CT: iodine quantification versus standard enhancement measurements. Eur Radiol 2013;23(8):2288–95.

31. Ascenti G, Krauss B, Mazziotti S, et al. Dual-energy computed tomography (DECT) in renal masses. Acad Radiol 2012;19(10):1186–93.

32. Ascenti G, Mazziotti S, Mileto A, et al. Dual-source dual-energy CT evaluation of complex cystic renal masses. Am J Roentgenol 2012;199(5):1026–34.

33. Brown CL, Hartman RP, Dzyubak OP, et al. Dual-energy CT iodine overlay technique for characterization of renal masses as cyst or solid: a phantom feasibility study. Eur Radiol 2009;19(5):1289–95.

34. Neville AM, Gupta RT, Miller CM, et al. Detection of renal lesion enhancement with dual-energy multidetector CT. Radiology 2011;259(1):173–83.

35. Liu X, Zhou J, Zeng M, et al. Homogeneous high attenuation renal cysts and solid masses-differentiation with single phase dual energy computed tomography. Clin Radiol 2013;68(4):e198–205. Available at: http://www.sciencedirect.com/science/article/pii/S0009926012005776.

36. Mileto A, Nelson RC, Samei E, et al. Impact of dual-energy multi–detector row CT with virtual monochromatic imaging on renal cyst pseudoenhancement: in vitro and in vivo study. Radiology 2014;272(3):767–76.

37. Jung DC, Oh YT, Kim MD, et al. Usefulness of the virtual monochromatic image in dual-energy spectral CT for decreasing renal cyst pseudoenhancement: a phantom study. Am J Roentgenol 2012;199(6):1316–9.

38. Manglaviti G, Tresoldi S, Guerrer CS, et al. In vivo evaluation of the chemical composition of urinary stones using dual-energy CT. Am J Roentgenol 2011;197(1):W76–83.

39. Ascenti G, Siragusa C, Racchiusa S, et al. Stone-targeted dual-energy CT: a new diagnostic approach to urinary calculosis. Am J Roentgenol 2010;195(4):953–8.

40. Stolzmann P, Kozomara M, Chuck N, et al. In vivo identification of uric acid stones with dual-energy CT: diagnostic performance evaluation in patients. Abdom Imaging 2010;35(5):629–35.

41. Jepperson MA, Cernigliaro JG, Sella D, et al. Dual-energy CT for the evaluation of urinary calculi: image interpretation, pitfalls and stone mimics. Clin Radiol 2013;68(12):e707–14.

42. Boland GW, Lee M, Gazelle GS, et al. Characterization of adrenal masses using unenhanced CT: an analysis of the CT literature. AJR Am J Roentgenol 1998;171(1):201–4.

43. Helck A, Hummel N, Meinel FG, et al. Can single-phase dual-energy CT reliably identify adrenal adenomas? Eur Radiol 2014;24(7):1636–42.

44. Gnannt R, Fischer M, Goetti R, et al. Dual-energy CT for characterization of the incidental adrenal mass: preliminary observations. Am J Roentgenol 2012; 198(1):138–44.

45. Kim YK, Park BK, Kim CK, et al. Adenoma characterization: adrenal protocol with dual-energy CT. Radiology 2013;267(1):155–63.

46. Botsikas D, Triponez F, Boudabbous S, et al. Incidental adrenal lesions detected on enhanced abdominal dual-energy CT: can the diagnostic workup be shortened by the implementation of virtual unenhanced images? Eur J Radiol 2014; 83(10):1746–51.

47. Marin D, Nelson RC, Samei E, et al. Hypervascular liver tumors: low tube voltage, high tube current multidetector CT during late hepatic arterial phase for detection—initial clinical experience. Radiology 2009;251(3):771–9.

48. Shuman WP, Green DE, Busey JM, et al. Dual-energy liver CT: effect of monochromatic imaging on lesion detection, conspicuity, and contrast-to-noise ratio of hypervascular lesions on late arterial phase. Am J Roentgenol 2014;203(3):601–6.

49. Robinson E, Babb J, Chandarana H, et al. Dual source dual energy MDCT: comparison of 80 kVp and weighted average 120 kVp data for conspicuity of hypo-vascular liver metastases. Invest Radiol 2010;45(7):413–8.

50. Patel BN, Thomas JV, Lockhart ME, et al. Single-source dual-energy spectral multidetector CT of pancreatic adenocarcinoma: optimization of energy level viewing significantly increases lesion contrast. Clin Radiol 2013;68(2):148–54.

51. McNamara MM, Little MD, Alexander LF, et al. Multi-reader evaluation of lesion conspicuity in small pancreatic adenocarcinomas: complimentary value of iodine material density and low keV simulated monoenergetic images using multiphasic rapid kVp-switching dual energy CT. Abdom Imaging 2015;40(5):1230–40.

52. Yamada Y, Jinzaki M, Tanami Y, et al. Virtual monochromatic spectral imaging for the evaluation of hypovascular hepatic metastases: the optimal monochromatic level with fast kilovoltage switching dual-energy computed tomography. Invest Radiol 2012;47(5):292–8.

53. Sudarski S, Apfaltrer P, Nance JW, et al. Objective and subjective image quality of liver parenchyma and hepatic metastases with virtual monoenergetic dual-source dual-energy CT reconstructions. Acad Radiol 2014;21(4):514–22.

54. Caruso D, De Cecco CN, Schoepf UJ, et al. Can dual-energy computed tomography improve visualization of hypoenhancing liver lesions in portal venous phase? Assessment of advanced image-based virtual monoenergetic images. Clin Imaging 2017;41(Supplement C):118–24.

Strategies to Improve Image Quality on Dual-Energy Computed Tomography

Bhavik N. Patel, MD, MBA[a],*, Daniele Marin, MD[b]

KEYWORDS

- Dual-energy CT • Image quality • Virtual monoenergetic images • Artifact • Metal

KEY POINTS

- Dual-energy computed tomography (DECT) is a promising modality that offers several advantages over conventional single-energy CT.
- Sources of potential image quality degradation may exist that are related to either the technical factors or the image reconstruction methods specific to DECT platform type.
- Familiarity with solutions to such potential sources of suboptimal image quality is crucial for routine clinical adoption of DECT.

INTRODUCTION

Dual-energy computed tomography (DECT) has gained much promise as a diagnostic modality. Through simultaneous (eg, dual-layer detector DECTs) and near-simultaneous (eg, single source, rapid kilovoltage-switching DECT [rsDECT] and dual-source DECT [dsDECT]) low- and high-energy acquisition, it offers several advantages and capabilities over conventional polychromatic images. These capabilities include material decomposition analysis (eg, iodine quantification), generation of material density images (**Fig. 1**), and reconstruction of virtual monoenergetic images (VMIs) across a wide x-ray energy range (ie, 40–190 keV).[1–3] VMIs have several advantages over conventional polychromatic images, including decreased susceptibility to beam hardening, improved image quality, and metal artifact reduction.[4–9] Moreover, VMIs at lower energy levels (eg, 50–60 keV) have increased iodine contrast as they approximate the K-edge of iodine, resulting in improved lesion conspicuity and vascular and parenchymal enhancement.[10] Such clinical value has led to widespread adoption of dual energy for several CT protocols across practices.[11] Although early momentum of rapid clinical adoption and use of DECT was plagued by image quality issues and noise, current DECT technology has allowed exceptional image quality and areas of improving it for certain niche applications (eg, metal artifact reduction). In this article, the authors review common sources of image-quality degradation that may exist because of the inherent dual-energy technology and acquisition and known strategies that overcome these limitations that have allowed routine usage of DECT in busy clinical practices. Based on the experience of the authors, this article focuses specifically on the rsDECT and dsDECT platforms.

Disclosure Statement: B.N. Patel: research support and consultant, GE Healthcare; D. Marin: research support, Siemens Healthcare.

[a] Division of Abdominal Imaging, Department of Radiology, Stanford University School of Medicine, 300 Pasteur Drive, H1307, Stanford, CA 94305, USA; [b] Division of Abdominal Imaging, Department of Radiology, Duke University, DUMC 3808, Durham, NC 27710, USA

* Corresponding author.

E-mail address: bhavikp@stanford.edu

Radiol Clin N Am 56 (2018) 641–647
https://doi.org/10.1016/j.rcl.2018.03.006

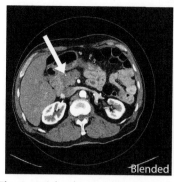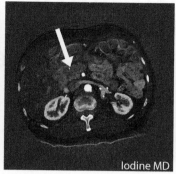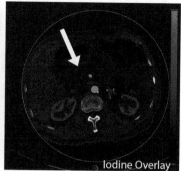

Fig. 1. Axial enhanced blended 120-kVp (50% tube A/50% tube B) equivalent image (*left*) shows a pancreatic head adenocarcinoma (*arrow*). Notice the increased lesion conspicuity on the iodine material density (MD) image (*middle*) and iodine color overlay image (*right*).

SPECTRAL SEPARATION

One of the major advantages of DECT is to allow quantitative compositional analysis of a given tissue, a task not possible with conventional attenuation measurements using single-energy polychromatic imaging. The CT number for a given voxel is related to the linear attenuation coefficient, which in turn is based on the atomic number of the elements, density, and the energy level.[12] For human tissue, 2 different elements with different densities may have similar attenuation at a given energy level. Consider, for example, tissues containing dense iodine or faint calcification, both of which may appear similar. However, with DECT, attenuation measurement at a second energy level would allow material differentiation.[1,2,12] The greater the degree of spectral separation of the low- and high-energy tube output used for dual-energy scanning, the greater the capability, reliability, and quality of material decomposition.[13] Traditionally, 80 kVp and 140 kVp commonly represented the low- and high-energy tube voltage settings, respectively, to achieve the spectral separation. This high and low energy selection affected image quality that necessitated a solution for both the rsDECT and dsDECT platforms.

Rapid-Kilovolt Switching Dual-Energy Computed Tomography

The second- and third-generation rsDECT scanners operate by using a single x-ray source that rapidly switches between 80 and 140 kVp during each rotation, with a fast switch time of 0.25 milliseconds. However, because of the significant tube ramp up and down between the high and low tube voltage, independent filtration and tube current modulation are not possible. Additionally, the rapid switching time between the high- and low-energy projections results in relatively decreased maximum x-ray flux.[2,12,14] Thus, without corrective strategies, each acquisition would result in images with poor quality attributed to photon starvation. In an effort to account for the aforementioned technical limitations, asymmetric sampling with 2 projections at the low tube voltage and one at the high tube voltage is acquired. This increase in sampling time allows the tube current-time product (milliampere) to be increased despite the lack of tube current modulation.[12] This increased sampling of the low tube voltage projection comes at a cost of associated increase in noise. To offset the noise, adaptive statistical iterative reconstruction techniques (ASIR and ASIR-V) are used.[2]

Dual-Source Dual-Energy Computed Tomography

Unlike the rsDECT, the dsDECT platforms are equipped with 2 x-ray sources and 2 x-ray detectors that have an angular offset. Because each tube is independent, tube current modulation and independent filtration is possible. The high-energy tube output can be filtered with a 0.4-mm tin (Sn) filter placed distal to the bowtie filter. This filtration results in a greater spectral separation between the low- and high-energy tube outputs.[13,15] This separation in turn translates to improved material decomposition. Using 80 kVp for the lower-energy tube output may potentially limit large patients from being scanned with DECT because of photon starvation. However, Sn filtration allows increasing the tube voltage for the larger tube A from 80 to 100 kVP for the second-generation dsDECT scanner or from 90 to 100 kVp for the third-generation scanner. Finally, the third-generation dsDECT scanner (ie, force) achieves a greater separation than the second-generation scanner by increasing the voltage setting of the larger tube A (ie, 150 Sn vs 140 Sn).

Another well-known potential technical source of image quality degradation of the dsDECT platform is the limited field of view (FOV) for scanning in dual-energy mode. Although the rsDECT allows scanning in dual-energy mode using the full 50-cm FOV, the dsDECT is limited based on the detector size of the smaller tube B (ie, 33-cm scan FOV for flash and 35-cm FOV for the force).[2,12] Anatomy outside of the dual-energy scan FOV is imaged with the lower voltage tube A. In order to preserve image quality for the anatomic area under study, the technologist must ensure patients are centered or positioned appropriately so that the relevant anatomy being scanned is covered within the dual-energy FOV (**Fig. 2**). Because of this FOV limitation, several institutions use a weight cutoff or a scout radiograph lateral diameter cutoff, though the exact cutoff threshold varies from institution to institution.[11]

VIRTUAL MONOENERGETIC IMAGES

VMIs may be synthesized from the dual-energy data sets, which simulate an ideal x-ray beam. VMIs offer several advantages over conventional polychromatic images, including decreased susceptibility to beam hardening, improved image quality, and metal artifact reduction.[4–9] VMIs are generated through basis material decomposition, and the approach differs depending on the platform used. For the dsDECT, an image-based method is used to reconstruct VMI from the low- and high-energy images. A projection-based method is used for the rsDECT platform in which VMI are created using projection domain basis material decomposition.[16] VMIs from 40 to 190 keV can be reconstructed in 1-keV increments.

In clinical practice, 70 to 75 keV is considered the single-energy 120-kVp polychromatic beam equivalent, as it has been validated as such with comparable attenuation values.[8,11] A high electron

volt may be used for metal artifact reduction and improve anatomic visualization that would otherwise be limited because of streak artifact. A low electron volt has the advantage of increased contrast, as it approximates the K-edge of iodine. This result, in turn, allows increased vascular and parenchymal contrast enhancement as well as lesion conspicuity, for both hypervascular and hypovascular lesions.[11] However, the clinical utility of a low electron volt VMI is limited because of a concomitants steep increase in noise and vulnerability to artifacts leading to image-quality degradation.[8,9,16]

To mitigate the noise associated with lower-energy VMI, a second-generation monoenergetic algorithm is used for the dsDECT image-based reconstruction of VMI.[17] This algorithm uses a spatial frequency-split technique recombining of the superior contrast signal from the low energy levels with the lower noise characteristics of the medium energy (ie, 70–75 keV) levels. Several studies have demonstrated optimal image quality and improved contrast-to-noise ratio of low electron volt VMI in various abdominal applications using this second-generation algorithm[18,19] (**Fig. 3**). For the rsDECT, noise from the lower-energy VMIs can be partially reduced using iterative reconstruction.[20]

METAL ARTIFACT REDUCTION

The presence of metal can cause significant artifact, which may impair the diagnostic task of the radiologist and thereby have significant clinical consequences. For example, consider a patient with bilateral hip prostheses and a history of rectal adenocarcinoma. The presence of metal may obscure the presence of regional nodal

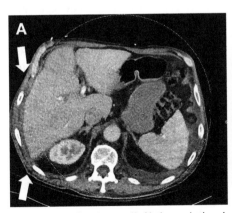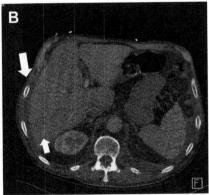

Fig. 2. (A) Axial enhanced CT image (*left*) through the abdomen scanned on a dsDECT shows a patient who is not centered within the dual-energy field-of-view (FOV) (denoted by *dotted circle*). As a result, there is decreased image contrast and degradation of image noise outside of this FOV (*arrows*). (B) Corresponding iodine overlay image (*right*) shows corresponding lack of iodine overlay outside of the dual-energy FOV (*long arrow*). As a consequence, part of the liver has been excluded from the dual-energy FOV (*short arrow*).

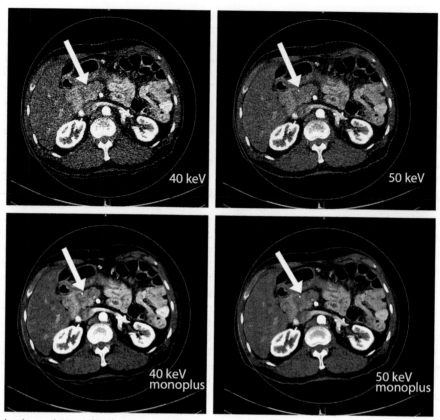

Fig. 3. Axial enhanced 40- and 50-keV images of the same patient from **Fig. 1** shows a pancreatic head adenocarcinoma. Note the increased contrast as well as noise (*top row*) of these low electron volt images when reconstructed using the first-generation reconstruction algorithm. When the second-generation algorithm (mono-plus) is used, note the substantial decrease in noise (*bottom row*).

metastases within the pelvis because of photon starvation and artifact secondary to the presence of metal.

VMIs at high energy levels (ie, 140 keV) can be used to reduce beam hardening and streak artifact thereby improving visualization of structures near or adjacent to metal.[16] However, as the VMI energy level increases, soft tissue contrast decreases. Additionally, high VMI, although allowing some improvement in image quality in the presence of metal, does not account for other sources of poor image quality, such as photon starvation and nonlinear partial volume averaging.[16,21] Thus, other iterative techniques are often required.[22]

Both the rsDECT and dsDECT have vendor-specific iterative metal artifact reduction (MAR) software that is compatible with dual-energy scanning. For the rsDECT gemstone spectral imaging MAR, metal segmentation and mask creation are performed using the high-kilovolt peak projection data. The metal-containing projection samples are removed from both the low- and high-kilovolt peak projection; through forward projection to estimate the missing samples from the segmented

images, final images are created by combining the estimated projections with the masked projections.[21,23] For the dsDECT, a relatively new iterative software algorithm has been developed (ie, iterative Metal Artifact Reduction [Siemens Healthcare, Forchheim, Germany]) that combines 2 prior algorithms, the normalized MAR (NMAR) and frequency-split MAR (FSMAR). IMAR simultaneously exploits the benefits of NMAR's ability to avoid artifacts that are tangential to high contrast objects and FSMAR's edge information preservation.[24]

Studies have shown the added benefit of MAR with dual-energy VMI compared with either method of metal artifact reduction alone[21,25] (**Fig. 4**).

FUTURE DIRECTIONS: MULTI-ENERGY COMPUTED TOMOGRAPHY

Spectral photon-counting CT (SPCCT) is an imaging modality that is currently under research and technological development and is being translated into clinical studies.[12,26–33] The important

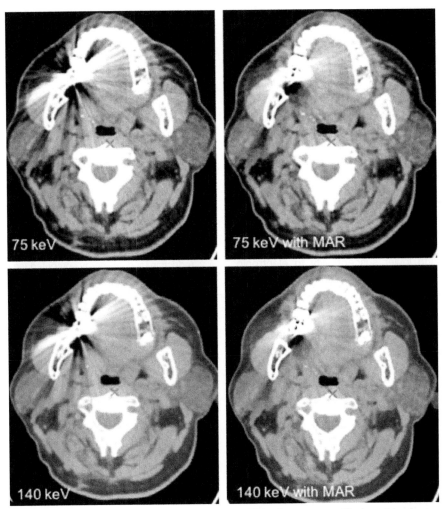

Fig. 4. Axial unenhanced CT images at the level of the mandible shows a metallic dental implant on the right. Note the interval decrease in metal streak artifact when using a high-energy VMI (ie, 140 keV). Metal artifact reduction (MAR) similarly improves image quality when used with the 75-keV image (*top right*). Note the incremental cumulative benefit when MAR is used with dual-energy metal artifact reduction methods (*bottom right*).

advantages of SPCCT, compared with current DECT technology, are based on the concept that incoming photons are counted and spectrally binned by analyzing the pulse amplitudes generated in a photon-counting detector. This technique could translate to improved image quality for multi-energy CT.

Photon-counting detectors use semiconductor materials, such as cadmium telluride, to directly convert individual x-ray photons into an electric signal pulse.[31,33] The energy deposited by each x-ray photon incident onto the photon-counting detectors generates electrical charges that will travel within the detector under the influence of a strong electrical field toward the anode and induce a pulse signal.[33] The amplitude of the pulse signal is proportional to the energy of the individual

incident photons, and photons of different energies contribute equally to the photon counts.[33] Therefore, photon-counting detectors discriminate the transmitted photons based on their energy and separate them into several energy bins.[12] Placing the energy bin boundaries close to the K-edge energies of different elements allows element-specific imaging (ie, K-edge imaging).[12,31] Ideally, the amplitude of the pulse signal should depend just on the photons with energy values within the range of the determined energy bin boundaries. In practice, physical effects, such as K-escape due to the photoelectric effect, Compton scattering, pulse pileup, detector polarization, charge sharing and trapping, may potentially impair the ideal separation of photons of different energies using photon-counting detectors.[31,33]

Using SPCCT, the K-edge absorption can be used to discriminate between different high-Z (atomic number) materials allowing multi-material quantification.[26–30] Additionally, one or more boundaries of the energy bins can be freely adjusted to match the K-edge of different contrast media, thus, allowing for dual-contrast agent imaging.[26,30] This imaging expands the possibilities of DECT, which is limited to the analysis of only 2 basis materials.[2,34]

Spectral CT imaging methods based on the photon-counting detectors (ie, K-edge and energy weighting imaging) proved to have similar or even higher image diagnostic quality in comparison with the conventional DECT imaging method.[35–38] The improvement in image quality can be related to several characteristics of photon counting detectors, including lower susceptibility to electronic noise, enhanced iodine contrast, the ability to weigh low-energy photons higher than high-energy photons, and decreased beam hardening and calcium blooming artifacts.[35,38] These benefits lead to better stability of CT numbers, lower image noise, higher contrast-to-noise properties, and, thus, improved dose efficiency.[35,37] This increase in contrast-to-noise ratio is particularly evident at higher tube potentials, which are necessary when imaging moderate to extremely large size patients, and may potentially allow for a reduction of the dose.[35]

Another advantage of photon-counting detectors is the smaller size of the pixel over the energy integrating detector.[33] This difference in size is due to the different way of structuring pixel in the 2 detectors. Although structuring pixel for conventional energy integrating detector requires a mechanical separation of the pixel, in photon-counting detectors pixels can be structured in a photolithographic process without the need of a mechanical separation to allowing for smaller pixel sizes. The smaller detector pixel size and the narrower photon-counting detector may lead to a superior spatial resolution of SPCCT images, defined by the Nyquist frequency of the sampling condition.[33,38,39]

SUMMARY

DECT technology has significantly improved with the latest third-generation scanners compared with initial first-generation scanners. In addition to improvement in workflow, a large component of the improvements have been secondary to developing solutions to improve image quality that otherwise might be limited secondary to inherent technical properties of the platforms and scanners. These solutions either come in the form of how the primary data are acquired or through improved VMI reconstruction algorithms, as examples.

REFERENCES

1. Coursey CA, Nelson RC, Boll DT, et al. Dual-energy multidetector CT: how does it work, what can it tell us, and when can we use it in abdominopelvic imaging? Radiographics 2010;30(4):1037–55.
2. Marin D, Boll DT, Mileto A, et al. State of the art: dual-energy CT of the abdomen. Radiology 2014;271(2):327–42.
3. Megibow AJ, Sahani D. Best practice: implementation and use of abdominal dual-energy CT in routine patient care. AJR Am J Roentgenol 2012;199(5 Suppl):S71–7.
4. Bamberg F, Dierks A, Nikolaou K, et al. Metal artifact reduction by dual energy computed tomography using monoenergetic extrapolation. Eur Radiol 2011;21(7):1424–9.
5. Dilmanian FA. Computed tomography with monochromatic X rays. Am J Physiol Imaging 1992;7(3–4):175–93.
6. Jung DC, Oh YT, Kim MD, et al. Usefulness of the virtual monochromatic image in dual-energy spectral CT for decreasing renal cyst pseudoenhancement: a phantom study. AJR Am J Roentgenol 2012;199(6):1316–9.
7. Lee MJ, Kim S, Lee SA, et al. Overcoming artifacts from metallic orthopedic implants at high-field-strength MR imaging and multi-detector CT. Radiographics 2007;27(3):791–803.
8. Matsumoto K, Jinzaki M, Tanami Y, et al. Virtual monochromatic spectral imaging with fast kilovoltage switching: improved image quality as compared with that obtained with conventional 120-kVp CT. Radiology 2011;259(1):257–62.
9. Yu L, Christner JA, Leng S, et al. Virtual monochromatic imaging in dual-source dual-energy CT: radiation dose and image quality. Med Phys 2011;38(12):6371–9.
10. Agrawal MD, Pinho DF, Kulkarni NM, et al. Oncologic applications of dual-energy CT in the abdomen. Radiographics 2014;34(3):589–612.
11. Patel BN, Alexander L, Allen B, et al. Dual-energy CT workflow: multi-institutional consensus on standardization of abdominopelvic MDCT protocols. Abdom Radiol (NY) 2017;42(3):676–87.
12. McCollough CH, Leng S, Yu L, et al. Dual- and multi-energy CT: principles, technical approaches, and clinical applications. Radiology 2015;276(3):637–53.
13. Krauss B, Grant KL, Schmidt BT, et al. The importance of spectral separation: an assessment of dual-energy spectral separation for quantitative ability and dose efficiency. Invest Radiol 2015;50(2):114–8.

14. Silva AC, Morse BG, Hara AK, et al. Dual-energy (spectral) CT: applications in abdominal imaging. Radiographics 2011;31(4):1031–46 [discussion: 1047–50].

15. Primak AN, Ramirez Giraldo JC, Liu X, et al. Improved dual-energy material discrimination for dual-source CT by means of additional spectral filtration. Med Phys 2009;36(4):1359–69.

16. Yu L, Leng S, McCollough CH. Dual-energy CT-based monochromatic imaging. AJR Am J Roentgenol 2012;199(5 Suppl):S9–15.

17. Grant KL, Flohr TG, Krauss B, et al. Assessment of an advanced image-based technique to calculate virtual monoenergetic computed tomographic images from a dual-energy examination to improve contrast-to-noise ratio in examinations using iodinated contrast media. Invest Radiol 2014; 49(9):586–92.

18. Bellini D, Gupta S, Ramirez-Giraldo JC, et al. Use of a noise optimized monoenergetic algorithm for patient-size independent selection of an optimal energy level during dual-energy CT of the pancreas. J Comput Assist Tomogr 2017;41(1):39–47.

19. Marin D, Ramirez-Giraldo JC, Gupta S, et al. Effect of a noise-optimized second-generation monoenergetic algorithm on image noise and conspicuity of hypervascular liver tumors: an in vitro and in vivo study. AJR Am J Roentgenol 2016;206(6):1222–32.

20. Zhao L, Winklhofer S, Yang Z, et al. Optimal adaptive statistical iterative reconstruction percentage in dual-energy monochromatic CT portal venography. Acad Radiol 2016;23(3):337–43.

21. Pessis E, Campagna R, Sverzut JM, et al. Virtual monochromatic spectral imaging with fast kilovoltage switching: reduction of metal artifacts at CT. Radiographics 2013;33(2):573–83.

22. Morsbach F, Bickelhaupt S, Wanner GA, et al. Reduction of metal artifacts from hip prostheses on CT images of the pelvis: value of iterative reconstructions. Radiology 2013;268(1):237–44.

23. Han SC, Chung YE, Lee YH, et al. Metal artifact reduction software used with abdominopelvic dual-energy CT of patients with metal hip prostheses: assessment of image quality and clinical feasibility. AJR Am J Roentgenol 2014;203(4):788–95.

24. Axente M, Paidi A, Von Eyben R, et al. Clinical evaluation of the iterative metal artifact reduction algorithm for CT simulation in radiotherapy. Med Phys 2015;42(3):1170–83.

25. Bongers MN, Schabel C, Thomas C, et al. Comparison and combination of dual-energy- and iterative-based metal artefact reduction on hip prosthesis and dental implants. PLoS One 2015;10(11): e0143584.

26. Cormode DP, Si-Mohamed S, Bar-Ness D, et al. Multicolor spectral photon-counting computed tomography: in vivo dual contrast imaging with a high count rate scanner. Sci Rep 2017;7(1):4784.

27. Ferrero A, Gutjahr R, Henning A, et al. Renal stone characterization using high resolution imaging mode on a photon counting detector CT system. Proc SPIE Int Soc Opt Eng 2017;10132 [pii: 101323J].

28. Kirkbride TE, Raja AY, Muller K, et al. Discrimination between calcium hydroxyapatite and calcium oxalate using multienergy spectral photon-counting CT. AJR Am J Roentgenol 2017;209(5):1088–92.

29. Leng S, Zhou W, Yu Z, et al. Spectral performance of a whole-body research photon counting detector CT: quantitative accuracy in derived image sets. Phys Med Biol 2017;62(17):7216–32.

30. Muenzel D, Bar-Ness D, Roessl E, et al. Spectral photon-counting CT: initial experience with dual-contrast agent K-edge colonography. Radiology 2017;283(3):723–8.

31. Schlomka JP, Roessl E, Dorscheid R, et al. Experimental feasibility of multi-energy photon-counting K-edge imaging in pre-clinical computed tomography. Phys Med Biol 2008;53(15):4031–47.

32. Shikhaliev PM. Computed tomography with energy-resolved detection: a feasibility study. Phys Med Biol 2008;53(5):1475–95.

33. Taguchi K, Iwanczyk JS. Vision 20/20: single photon counting x-ray detectors in medical imaging. Med Phys 2013;40(10):100901.

34. Mileto A, Marin D. Dual-energy computed tomography in genitourinary imaging. Radiol Clin North Am 2017;55(2):373–91.

35. Gutjahr R, Halaweish AF, Yu Z, et al. Human imaging with photon counting-based computed tomography at clinical dose levels: contrast-to-noise ratio and cadaver studies. Invest Radiol 2016;51(7):421–9.

36. Pourmorteza A, Symons R, Sandfort V, et al. Abdominal imaging with contrast-enhanced photon-counting CT: first human experience. Radiology 2016; 279(1):239–45.

37. Symons R, Pourmorteza A, Sandfort V, et al. Feasibility of dose-reduced chest CT with photon-counting detectors: initial results in humans. Radiology 2017; 285(3):980–9.

38. Yu Z, Leng S, Jorgensen SM, et al. Evaluation of conventional imaging performance in a research whole-body CT system with a photon-counting detector array. Phys Med Biol 2016;61(4):1572–95.

39. Leng S, Gutjahr R, Ferrero A, et al. Ultra-high spatial resolution, multi-energy CT using photon counting detector technology. Proc SPIE Int Soc Opt Eng 2017;10132 [pii:101320Y].

Printed and bound by CPI Group (UK) Ltd, Croydon, CR0 4YY

08/05/2025

01864713-0016